Emotional Intelligence - A resource for nurses

Carlos Vilela

Emotional Intelligence - A resource for nurses

Contributions to the management, training and development of emotional skills

ScienciaScripts

Cover image: www.ingimage.com

This book is a translation from the original published under ISBN 978-613-9-69450-1.

Publisher:
Sciencia Scripts
is a trademark of
Dodo Books Indian Ocean Ltd. and OmniScriptum S.R.L publishing group

120 High Road, East Finchley, London, N2 9ED, United Kingdom
Str. Armeneasca 28/1, office 1, Chisinau MD-2012, Republic of Moldova, Europe

ISBN: 978-620-7-21333-7

Table of contents:

I dedicate this book to you,

To my mother, Albertina, my father, Francisco,
and the loves of my life, Cristina and Carolina.

Thank you for the emotional balance you give me.

Thanks

To my Professors, posthumously, Professor James Stover Taylor and Professor Rui Santiago, for sharing all their knowledge with me.

To the nurses who contributed to the expansion of knowledge in this area.

To the Nursing School of Porto, which provides the best conditions for my professional development.

To Professor Augusta Veiga-Branco, mentor of the scale used in the research, for her advice and friendship.

To Professors: Maria de Lourdes Machado-Taylor, Célia Santos, Paulino Sousa, Paulo Parente, Ana Leonor Ribeiro, Alexandrina Cardoso, Alice Brito and Paulo Puga Machado, for all their support and encouragement.

To my friends: Justino, Pedro, André, Miguel and Américo, whom I still don't know how to repay for their friendship and the time they dedicate to me...

To my family, especially my brothers.

To many others who, directly or indirectly, supported the realization of this project.

Foreword

The students really wanted to learn. But what did I have to teach them? (...) What I knew best was that we are passengers, we are instants diluted in centuries of wills and destinies.

José Luís Peixoto. 2011. Abraco. p 358

Starting a Foreword is not an easy task. A preface is a face of. A preface is the face. The first image. What you want to make known as a first impression. In one word. In a single paragraph. Short, expressive and full of content.

And from this perspective, this book is about presenting self-learning - as real learning should be - from an empirical and insightful route, in the act of learning how to learn. In this case, learning the Emotional Competence of Nurses. It was a courageous task. Because it was initiatory, innovative and little explored, particularly in this working reality in Portugal.

At the time, common sense had looked curiously at this concept of Emotional Competence, in a tenuous and distant way, and rooted in the knowledge and understanding of what it understood as feelings, rather than emotions. And this concept was understood as a set of skills and normal aspects of development that would be useful to human beings in understanding themselves and others, necessary for empathy and relationships in general.

Thus, it was assumed that there were positive and negative emotions in life, with the former reserving the space of preference and desire to be experienced, and the latter, and by opposition, the space of repudiation, withdrawal and impediment to their experience. It was a practical example that anger would be a reaction to external aggression and would serve much more to repel aggression than for self-protection. What's more, from this perspective at the end of the 20th century, fear was assumed to be much more of a response to danger or mournful strangeness than an innate *arousal,* with the physiological effect of enhancing our attention and our senses in general, to guide and promote human reactions in order to manage and cope with the situation. The closest concept, because it was the most popular and socially presented - in fact the concept from which Emotional Competence originated - was known in the literature as Emotional Intelligence. And all this wealth of knowledge was thus transported to the field of work. In a field of work such as nursing, where the caring aspects, shaped by emotions, promote the acts of caring in a lively and dynamic way.

A field of work where yoga has real meaning

In fact, it was with great pertinence that an increasing number of nurses realized the added value of knowledge and the necessary applicability of Emotional Competence *skills* in the world of nursing work. Regardless of the type of pathology, age, social or economic status, nurses needed to establish what Cari Rogers conceived of as a therapeutic relationship with patients, whose interaction, according to the author, emerges from empathy, congruence and transparency.

In one way or another, a problem was felt and identified for the emotional climate of nursing care. How would it be possible to put concepts such as transparency, congruence... into practice in a training culture where emotions were much more the target of repression, suppression, than expression?

And the fact is that emotional suppression was educationally and culturally legitimized. We had all learned that emotional suppression was socially correct and useful, to avoid relational and social constraints. In one way or another, caring, in its most deeply genuine conception, needed to access what was most deeply genuine in the human. And, progressively, it was also realized that people oriented towards controlling or even suppressing their emotions (perceived as negative, inadequate) in order to ward off conflicts or discomfort in themselves, could inappropriately trigger somatizations and false concealment of problems which, as an indirect consequence, would result in less good for everyone involved (Gross & Levenson, 1997), but more precisely for users and patients.

It was in the 1980s, with Howard Gardner's concept of Multiple Intelligences, that the view of what is now known as *soft skills* expanded, reflecting on how the monolithic model of intelligence would make less sense than the concept of a multiplicity of areas of intelligibility, and in these the component of intra- and inter-relationship. Time progressed bringing new awakenings and concepts, and at the end of the 1980s, Peter Salovey and John Mayor published the concept that Goleman would have put into common sense, in a more expansive and broader way: Emotional Intelligence as a concept and its respective capacities, was largely the subject of the expectant curiosity of educators and teachers, as a new space for thinking about and understanding the human being.

In fact, since the 1990s, the literature has been expressing these realities more and more frequently. From the results of successive studies, we have all learned and become aware of how emotions should be taken into account, and their added value as a guide to and in cognition: in other words, more in the sense of managing them and not suppressing them.

The authors who have taken it upon themselves over time to explore this issue (Salovey & Mayer, 1990, 1994, 1999; Goleman, 1995, 1999; Bar-On, 1990; Boyatzis, Goleman, & Rhee, 1999; Saarni, 1999, 2000, 2007, 2011; Bisquerra, 1999, 2001; Veiga-Branco, 1995, 2000, 2002, 2011; Cassidy, 1994), it has become clear that emotionally competent people give themselves space and time to feel their emotions and learn to manage them so that they can express them in a way that suits the situation, their own needs and the needs of others. This aspect has become relevant in all fields of work and applicable to all age groups throughout the life *continuum*, not only in health but also in education (Reiff, Hatzes, Bramel, & Gibbon, 2001; Petrides, Frederickson, & Furnham, 2004).

In fact, the watchword has become: don't suppress your emotions, reactions or communicate your feelings (Thompson, 1991). The theoretical concept that emerged with Emotional Intelligence and Emotional Competence was precisely to give oneself personal space to recognize the emotions in oneself, to learn to manage these energies and to manage them in an appropriate way to make decisions and to be exposed to others, in order to improve relationships.

In this working context, it was understood and felt to be essential that learning the dimensions of Emotional Competence, such as recognizing one's emotions in the body and managing these activations, could make human beings better able to understand themselves and others, phenomena which, in symbiosis, are understood to promote health (Ciarrochi, Scott, Deane, & Heaven, 2003). This phenomenon alone could establish a physiology of inner harmony, promoting *normal* relationships between the subject and the world, avoiding stress and anguish, which would otherwise result from emotional suppression. Caring for frail people has made it clear that emotions that are considered negative, uncomfortable and inadequate are less likely to be expressed and recognized. It became easier to understand that the possibility of educating emotions, in the sense of acquiring a reasonable level of Emotional Competence, was an educational hypothesis that presented a more salutogenic understanding of human behavior. And it was along this path of new concepts and understandings that some professionals in educational and care settings began to explore a curious path of research and understanding, in order to recognize the actors in the fields of care work, where these skills were and continue to be assumed as essential. And it was on this journey of thinking about the act of caring in nursing that this trainer of nurses became an author!

From the author...

And suddenly this kid, who I think I know so well, transmutes into someone else, who is out of this world (...)
he's gone to the planet of Music, and it's as if nothing else can reach him or distract him. It's funny to see
him like that, in another dimension, because I feel it myself.

Miguel de Sousa Tavares (2014) You can't find what you're looking for, p 80

At first I had more teachers and fewer students. Then I had fewer and fewer teachers and more students... then I had followers... and over time, these followers took on their own expectations, creating and responding to new ideas, thinking their own thoughts, writing and defending those thoughts in thesis. and this is probably where they emerged, with the status of those who know what they're talking about, and became authors.

This incredible wave of meandering lives is itself a life. And it is in these meanderings that the new emerges, as the useful, the essential. It is therefore in this context that the author emerges. It happened more or less unexpectedly. In my life, as in Miguel Sousa Tavares', it seems that I don't find what I'm looking for either. On the contrary, it seems that it is those who seek me who find me. And Carlos Vilela sought me and found me! And what was he really looking for?

My work on Emotional Competence is based on the modified concepts of Goleman's (1995, 1999) mixed model of EI, on the one hand, and Saarni's (1990, 1995, 1997) and Bisquerra's (2000, 2003) concept of Emotional Competence, on the other. This modification emerged from the perception of the added value of Emotional Competence, based on what Goleman explores in Notes (1999, p 341), assuming that the expression "emotional competence" includes both social and emotional competences, clarifying that "*an emotional competence is a learned ability, (...) that results in outstanding performance at work*" (1999, p 33), where he pointed out that: "*Our Emotional Intelligence determines our potential to learn practical skills (.) Our emotional competence shows to what extent, we translate this potential into professional skills*". Thus, it was only later that I assumed (Veiga-Branco, 2005, p 171) that

"*E.C. exists when someone reaches a desired level of achievement*", a phenomenon which, in terms of after-the-fact, can only be appreciated simultaneously or after the display of behaviors and/or attitudes, through observation, or through the memories expressed by the performers or observers.

Thus, based on these authors as a theoretical framework, I developed a mixed and multifactorial model of E.C. (Veiga-Branco, 2005), which in order to understand it - with the object of study being the recognition of an E.C. profile -I created a data collection instrument: the Veiga Branco Scale of Emotional Intelligence Capacities (EVBCIE) (Veiga Branco, 2000, 2004, 2005, 2007), which was later reformulated into the current Veiga Scale of Emotional Competence (EVCE) (Veiga Branco, 2011, 2012). It was at this point that Carlos Vilela met me. He was looking for the EVBCIE to apply to a sample of nurses during his Master's thesis! And it is from this meeting of routes that the thesis emerged and the feeling of trust and solidarity that continues today. It is for these reasons that I am writing this Preface. It's as simple as that.

From an Investigation to the Paradigm of a Profession...

It is not possible to know and understand a reality without discovering it... it is essential that we are humble enough to accept that without scientific evidence, everything we say is just a set of opinions. And that's exactly why this work has brought a slice of that evidence to the world of nursing care! It has brought to the practical field a profile of *soft skills,* which are now known, reflected on, and which, from reflection, can help these or other professionals, how they can and should develop these skills!

In fact, the work presented in this book makes it clear how nurses perceive and feel about their Emotional Competence skills profile. But this is not the most important thing. The essential added value is that this author has identified, in a methodological and scientific manner, the image of the Emotional Competence profile that nurses construct and how they construct it, in order to apply their own learning in this relational field.

This work leads the health workforce to think about the need to know, believe, express and put into practice that it is not appropriate for emotional capital to be avoided through fear of triggering some "negative" emotion or reaction on the part of the other person.

The study reflects an insightful reality that makes clear the essential importance of human development in harmony, based on an economy of human emotional resources, which, once identified and managed, constitute a deep and strong real capital: emotional thinking and the emotional capital that drives our behaviors, and how they can be managed in order to achieve our goals.

This is where this work is important and relevant.

For nursing. For health. For life.

Maria Augusta Romao da Veiga Branco,

Coordinating Professor of the School of Health of the Polytechnic Institute of Braganca

PRESENTATION

The body of this text is basically divided into three parts. In the first, the theoretical background, a brief theoretical exposition is offered, where we hope to provide a general and brief knowledge of what Emotional Intelligence (EI) is, the concepts associated with it, as well as a measuring instrument that measures Emotional Intelligence abilities - the Veiga Branco Scale of Emotional Intelligence Abilities (EVB-CIE).

Secondly, the first research in Portugal into emotional intelligence (EI) in nursing professionals is presented. It will describe: the assumptions underlying the exploratory study; the methodological options; the development of the research and its main results. It will also present how the EVB-CIE scale was validated in a sample of 214 nurses from an EPE hospital, using principal component factorial analysis. A profile of EI is presented which corresponds to the nurses' perception of their abilities and overall EI. We also studied: some variables that seem to influence factors, skills and EI; the correlations between them and, finally, the explanatory variables of EI.

At the end of the book, and on the assumption that emotional intelligence skills are relevant to the professional practice of nurses, the author wishes to gather some data of interest for improving the training and management processes of nurses, as well as raising awareness of the usefulness of this type of intelligence in their lives and in that of organizations.

By the author's choice, this book was written under the old spelling agreement.

PRELIMINARY CONSIDERATIONS

Optimizing professional performance is inseparable from people's ability to recognize and control their emotions. People must be understood as the core of any organization, which is why the interest in and study of emotions is gaining more and more allies.

The influence of emotions in countless areas of human existence and activity is now recognized as a structuring dimension of people's personal and professional lives. Nowadays, the "best" are also distinguished by their self-confidence, self-control and integrity, as well as their ability to communicate, influence, put themselves in other people's shoes and adapt to change. In fact, whatever the professional activity, it is not enough to be endowed with cognitive intelligence or to be technically good. The evidence points to the need to develop some skills that are not exclusively cognitive, such as creativity, flexibility, aptitude, a spirit of mutual help and knowing how to be (Goleman, 2000, 2003; Salovey, Mayer and Caruso, 2002).

Emotional intelligence (EI) is not a new concept. It is based on a long history of research and the formulation of theories about social and personal behavior. Concerns about these issues have given rise to the development of various studies. In the last century, from the early 1990s onwards, the discussion around EI took shape. According to Goleman (2003), in this decade, Peter Salovey and John Mayer were the first researchers to develop scientific studies on this subject. Daniel Goleman sparked greater interest when he published *Emotional Intelligence* in different languages in 1995. This author presents an innovative idea: that you can be successful in life without having a brilliant career or academic background.

Assuming that the human factor is a central element of an organization's culture, there is a great need to deepen knowledge that helps to understand and organize human resources in their emotional components. The Ministry of Health, in a document on nursing education (Portugal. Ministério da Saúde, 2000), states that the aim in training future nursing professionals is to prepare them for a high level of adaptability to new professional situations, which will relentlessly arise during their career.

In 2003, the European Parliament referred to the need to recognize psychological harassment as an occupational health risk (cited by Fornés et al., 2004). Fornés et al. (2004) point out that psychological harassment is an increasingly frequent phenomenon in the workplace, affecting around 10% of workers in Europe. Issues such as isolation, personal humiliation, criticism, distortions in communication and professional discredit (including acts that attempt to demean professionally), are aspects that progressively isolate a professional from the rest of the team and affect their balance and, consequently, their commitment and professional performance. According to Queirós (2004; In Branco, 2004b, p.13):

> "Work-related stress is a concern that began in the 1980s and has been growing ever since. It is now considered a serious problem, as numerous psychological and/or physiological complaints are responsible for huge losses in productivity at work. In October 2002, during the European Week against Stress at Work, several studies were published stating that 50% of sick leave in the European Union is due to stress, and that work-related stress affects all professional classes."

Nursing is one of the professions that is particularly vulnerable to this phenomenon, being exposed to a wide range of sources of stress that can disrupt the well-being of these professionals. By observing their day-to-day work, we can easily identify some of the sources that trigger stress in nurses: The Ministry of Health's failure to value the profession and their own career; the lack of recognition of their social mandate by other professional groups and society itself; the often scarce material and human resources available, which compromise the quality of their performance; working hours, which are almost always rotating and uncertain; psychological factors related to contact with patients in great pain; professional risks related to safety and hygiene in the workplace, which are not always guaranteed by institutions and professionals; increasingly precarious contractual conditions; the need to make decisions quickly, interacting with a wide range of people and professionals; and, apart from anything else, contact with citizens with the most diverse characteristics, problems and illnesses. It is therefore extremely important to identify these sources of stress in order to define strategies to reduce their impact on this professional group.

Today, the notion that people are the driving force behind organizations is unavoidable. This is why modern societies are faced with the challenge of acquiring, developing and managing new professional skills - emotional skills. The operationalization of this challenge essentially involves, on the one hand, knowing the reality that interferes with the professional's day-to-day life, namely the way in which they experience their emotions, and, on the other, involving, listening to, stimulating and channelling their potential.

Nurses are service providers - essentially *care* providers - who, in the course of their practice, "produce" emotions, reactions and feelings. Given this, it makes sense to know and analyze the variables that influence their behavior and attitudes. They are professionals whose job requires them to know and control the management of their own emotions, as well as those of the people they work with (doctors, medical assistants, social workers, psychologists, managers and even the citizen/user themselves). According to Colell Brunet et al. (2004), the first step towards improving the training of health professionals in general, and nursing professionals in particular, is to get to know their attitudes and investigate their own emotions.

After reviewing the literature, and in view of the proposals made by various authors dedicated to the area of EI, it was considered necessary to choose a theoretical model that would help to conduct the study on the subject. The author who made it most feasible to transpose the problem of EI to the professional field of nursing was Daniel Goleman (2000, 2003). This psychologist, author of various works and research in this area of knowledge, continued and innovated the work of other researchers over many years, increasing the body of knowledge in this area.

Thus, his model emerges as the main reference for this book and the research that will be presented. It seemed a challenge to find out what EI skills nurses possess and, from there, to build knowledge that would contribute to the definition of development, training, management and selection strategies for these health professionals.

Our interest in studying the management of emotions and their impact on clinical nursing practice has been a constant in our journey. In fact, it has long been a concern that we would like to explore. Thus, the lack of literature and research on nursing professionals in Portugal is the main motivation for this publication. The object of analysis here is the emotional intelligence skills of nurses in the hospital context.

By getting to know the characteristics of nurses' Emotional Intelligence (also referred to by some authors as emotional competence [Goleman, 2000, 2003; Branco, 2004b]), we are encouraging reflection and intervention in order to enhance the development of emotional capacities in the professional nursing group, thus hoping to make a valid contribution to the management and training of these human resources.

PART I

THE CONTOURS OF INTELLIGENCE
EMOTIONAL

This part of the book provides a theoretical review of the concepts inherent in emotional intelligence, based essentially on Goleman's (2000, 2003) conceptualization. It focuses on some of the neurological factors that influence EI, namely the open circuit of emotions, which mean that EI abilities can be cultivated and strengthened throughout life, both at an individual and group level. The approach to the importance of EI for people's personal and professional lives is complemented by the presentation of the adaptation of a scale to measure nurses' EI abilities.

Chapter 1

1 - THE GENESIS OF THE CONCEPT

The notion that emotional intelligence (EI) is important for individual work is not new. But only recently has research begun to show that it is crucial for organizational success. This chapter will review the concept of EI, considering the views of various authors, particularly Daniel Goleman (2000, 2003) - the most cited researcher who serves as a model in our study.

In 1995, Goleman defined the concept of emotional intelligence (EI) as: "(...) the ability to motivate oneself and persist despite frustrations; to control impulses and delay rewards; to regulate one's own mood and prevent discouragement from overwhelming one's thinking; to feel empathy and hope" (Goleman, 2003, p.54). Later, in 1998, the author reformulated his definition by saying that EI is: "(...) the ability to recognize our feelings and those of others, to motivate ourselves and to manage emotions well in ourselves and in our relationships" (Goleman, 2000, p.323). EI is not merely about being nice. At times, it may even require not being nice and, for example, confronting someone openly with an unpleasant truth. This idea does not mean giving free rein to feelings, letting them flow, but rather allowing feelings to be managed in such a way that they can be expressed appropriately and effectively (Goleman, 2000).

In the view of Hedlund and Sternberg (2000), one of the limitations of Goleman's definition is that he tries to take away as much value as possible from the intelligence quotient (IQ). In this circumstance, Goleman (2000) states that EI abilities are more important than IQ for people's success. However, in his writings, he does not ignore the importance of both types of intelligence for personal and organizational development (Goleman, 2000, 2003).

According to Mayer and Salovey (1997, cited by Salovey, Mayer and Caruso, 2002), EI represents the ability to perceive and express emotions, achieving and/or generating feelings that facilitate cognitive activities and adaptive actions, the ability to regulate one's own emotions and those of others. In other words, EI represents the ability to competently process emotion information and use it to guide cognitive activities, such as problem-solving and focusing energy on desired behaviors.

For Salovey and Sluyter (1999), the concept of EI is underpinned by a set of capabilities, which can be approached in a compartmentalized way. Like Goleman (2000), the authors also refer to the concept of emotional competence - which occurs when a person reaches the desired level of achievement in a particular action (Salovey and Sluyter, 1999). These authors define EI as the core ability to reason with emotion and thus learn about emotion or the information it conveys.

Bellack (1999), wondering what exactly emotional intelligence is, completes the definition of the concept by saying that it encompasses personal competence (i.e. the ability to manage oneself) and social competence (i.e. the ability to relate to others). Personal competence involves self-awareness, self-regulation and motivation. It is reflected in certain characteristics: having self-confidence, knowing one's strengths and limits, having self-control of emotions, being trustworthy, being flexible, being comfortable with new ideas and change, taking initiative, being able to lead, respecting commitments, being optimistic, justifying one's own performance and giving one's best.

Somewhat differently from Goleman, Mayer and Salovey (1997, cited by Salovey, Mayer and Caruso, 2002 and Bueno and Primi, 2003) define the concept of EI as the ability to perceive, evaluate and express emotions accurately; the ability to access and/or generate feelings that facilitate thinking; the ability to understand emotions and emotional knowledge; the ability to regulate emotions promoting emotional and intellectual growth.

In general, the concepts presented by the various authors have common points that do not contradict each other (Salovey, Mayer and Caruso, 2002; Goleman, 2000, 2003; Shutte et al., 1998, 2001, cited by Branco, 2005). Goleman (2003) argues peremptorily that personal skills related to EI are important for success in various areas of life, particularly in work performance. He also says that academic intelligence has very little to do with emotional life, so that "people with a high IQ can turn out to be terrible pilots of their private lives" (Goleman, 2003, p.54). Unlike IQ, which changes little after adolescence, EI is assimilated and continues to develop throughout life, as we learn from our experiences and motivate ourselves to improve empathy and social skills. The author uses an elucidating word to define this growth in EI - "maturity" (Goleman, 2000, p.15).

1.1 - CONCEPTUAL DEVELOPMENT

A brief historical review of the concept, based on some of the authors who have contributed most to its evolution, shows that there is a long tradition of looking for links between the development of non-cognitive factors and people's success in their personal lives and in the workplace. Over the decades, various names have been used, some vague, ranging from "character" and "personality" to "personal qualities" and "competence" (Goleman, 2000, p.12). In the 1990s, a more precise understanding of these human talents and a new name for them finally emerged - "Emotional Intelligence" (Idem and Ibidem; Salovey, Mayer and Caruso, 2002). For some years now, this term has been used by various psychologists seeking to understand what an intelligent person really is.

According to Cherniss (2000), one of the first researchers to write on the subject was Robert

Thorndike who, at the end of the 1930s, tried to define the concept of *social intelligence*. In 1940, David Wechsler (cited by Cherniss, 2000) also referred to *non-intellective abilities* as essential for adaptation and success in life and, in the same year, under Hemphill's direction, *Ohio State Leadership Studies* listed some important social and emotional skills for good leadership, such as: communication skills, sensitivity, initiative and interpersonal relationships, which were tested in the private sector in 1956 (Cherniss, 2000). Unfortunately, the work of these pioneers was forgotten until 1983, when Howard Gardner revived the notion of *multiple intelligence*, arguing that *intrapersonal and interpersonal intelligences* were important for defining the type of intelligence typically assessed by IQ tests (Cherniss, 2000; Salovey, Mayer and Caruso, 2002). In the early 1980s, Reuven Bar-On used the abbreviation EQ (emotional quotient) for the first time to refer to EI abilities (Goleman, 2000).

According to Salovey, Mayer and Caruso (2002), it was Mowrer (1960) who first stated that emotions cannot be placed in opposition to intelligence (IQ). Later, Payne (1983/1986) used the term in an unpublished dissertation. Furthermore, a framework for emotional intelligence and suggestions for its measurement were described in two articles published in 1990 by Mayer, DiPaolo and Salovey (cited by Salovey, Mayer and Caruso, 2002).

In 1990, two psychologists, Peter Salovey and John Mayer first described the term emotional intelligence (EI) and became interested in its non-cognitive aspects (Salovey and Mayer, 1990; Cit by Vitello- Cicciu, 2003). These authors described it as a form of social intelligence that involves the ability to control the feelings and emotions of oneself or others, using information about emotion to achieve better thoughts and actions (Cherniss, 2000; Salovey, Mayer and Caruso, 2002). Originally, these scholars concluded that EI consisted of three mental processes: - evaluating and expressing emotions in oneself and others; - regulating one's own emotions and those of others; and - using emotions by adapting them to different situations. In 1997, EI was extended to four mental abilities: - identifying emotions, - integrating emotions into thought processes, - understanding emotions and - dealing with emotions (Mayer and Salovey, 1997). From then on, they began a research program with the intention of developing valid ways of measuring EI and exploring its meaning, developing several studies in which they linked certain personal characteristics with the ability to respond flexibly to change and the construction of social support networks (Cherniss, 2000).

Daniel Goleman, aware of the work of these authors, went ahead with the first edition of his book *Emotional Intelligence*, published in 1995, becoming one of the leading experts in the field. Goleman has written in the *New York Times* about the brain and behavioral sciences. He was trained by several Harvard psychologists, including David McClelland, who belonged to a group of researchers who were interested in small traditional tests of cognitive intelligence and their relationship to success factors in life (Goleman, 2000). What Goleman did was to compile and study the existing data, giving the subject a scientific character, substantiating the concepts developed by the previous authors with empirical data (Salovey, Mayer and Caruso, 2002). Goleman is co-director of the *Consortium for Social and Emotional Learning in the Workplace,* dedicated to identifying the best practices for developing EI skills (Goleman, 2000).

In the same year, a few months before Goleman's book was published in the United States, Roberto Lira Miranda published *Beyond Emotional Intelligence: Integral Use of Brain Skills in Learning, Work and Life*, the fruit of his research work since 1992 in top companies (Miranda, 2003). In this book, the author points out that both science and common sense recognize that human beings have underused mental capacities (Miranda, 2003). Based on this assumption, he presents an enlightening dissertation on the scientifically based theories of human intelligence and brain abilities. Miranda (2003) seems to want to reinforce what other scientists and philosophers once thought, arguing that man uses no more than twenty percent of his intellectual and cerebral potential. Thus, he addresses issues related to the importance of the full use of brain skills in the performance of all activities, highlighting: teaching/learning processes; raising children; communication; coexistence and teamwork; leadership at work and in the family and business management.

1.2 - EMOTIONAL INTELLIGENCE VS. COGNITIVE INTELLIGENCE

Goleman (2000), as a student at Harvard and then as a professor, was part of one of the first challenges to the IQ mystique. The author points out that there is a false - but widespread - notion that what determines success is intellect alone. On the other hand, he points out that IQ is second only to EI in determining outstanding professional performance and that IQ alone is not a good indicator of job performance.

Cherniss (2000) refers to authors such as Hunter, Hunter and Sternberg, who have tried to quantify the importance of IQ in work environments, with some studies attributing very low values to the relationship, in the order of four percent. The same author also adds that social and emotional skills are four times more important than IQ in determining professional success and prestige (Idem). According to Goleman, Boyatzis and McKee (2002), EI can be more important in people's lives than cognitive intelligence itself (assessed by IQ). They go on to say that empathy and self-awareness are much more relevant to emotional competence than cognitive intelligence (Idem; Salovey, Mayer and Caruso, 2002; Goleman, 2003).

In an analysis of data from around 500 competency models, carried out in large companies, health institutions, universities, government departments and a religious order (all American), Goleman, Boyatzis and McKee (2002) concluded that purely cognitive competencies help, but EI competencies help much more in promoting exceptional performance. In these studies, the authors compared the best top leaders with average performers at the same hierarchical level and found that cognitive competencies are the skills a leader needs in order to perform at an average level. EI competencies make up the vast majority of capabilities that have a differentiating character (Idem).

For his part, Goleman (2000) points out that the world is full of men and women with good educational qualifications who were once promising, but who have since stagnated in their careers or, worse still, failed to achieve the career they wanted because of their lack of EI. In the American context, in a more or less explicit way, EI skills are taken into account for the recruitment and promotion of employees in companies. In a national survey in the United States, which asked what employers were looking for in entry-level workers, specific technical skills proved to be less important than the underlying ability to learn through training courses provided by the employer. It should be noted that of the desired characteristics, only one was academic - competence in reading, writing and mathematics (Carnevale et al., cited by Goleman, 2000). According to these authors, technical skills follow a list of preferences:

- Listening and oral communication skills;
- Ability to adapt and respond creatively to setbacks and obstacles;
- Self-determination, confidence, motivation for goal-oriented work, willingness to progress in your career and take pride in your commitments;
- Efficiency in groups and interpersonal relationships, ability to cooperate and work

as part of a team, negotiating skills in disagreements.
- Efficiency in organization, willingness to contribute, leadership potential.

Dowd and Liedtka (cited by Goleman, 2000, p.21) revealed a similar list in a study on what companies look for in an MBA (Master of Business Administration) holder. The three most sought-after skills are the ability to communicate, interpersonal skills and initiative. These authors also refer to the words of Jill Fadule, director of admissions and financial assistant at Harvard University's School of Management, who says that empathy, the ability to approach issues from various perspectives, bonding and cooperation are among the skills that the School looks for in applicants (Goleman, 2000).

Another example is given by Goleman (2000), in a study of Harvard graduates (in the fields of law, medicine, teaching and management and administration). This study revealed that entrance exam scores - based on IQ - had little or no correlation with eventual career success. It also concluded that IQ has the lowest ability to predict success among the group of people who are intelligent enough to master the most demanding cognitive areas and that the value of EI for success increases the higher the intelligence barriers to entry into a given area. Reinforcing this idea, the author argues that emotional climate influences cognitive intelligence, considering the exclusive contribution of IQ to success in life and work to be reductive, i.e. both types of intelligence influence the way we lead our lives, making it important to find a balance between these two forms of intelligence, since the mind cannot function perfectly without EI (Goleman, 2003).

1.3 - NEUROLOGY OF EMOTIONS

According to Goleman (2000), the prefrontal region (the executive center of the brain) is where *working memory* resides, i.e. the ability to pay attention and keep important information in mind, and is vital for comprehension and understanding, planning and decision-making, reasoning and learning. Personal skills and leadership are also related to the structure of the brain - the *limbic brain* - through the transmission of emotional impulses between the vast circuits that exist between the amygdalae and the prefrontal area (Goleman, Boyatzis and McKee, 2002).

When the mind is calm, working memory functions are at their maximum, but when emergency situations arise, the brain switches to a self-protective mode, withdrawing resources from working memory and allocating them to other parts of the brain to keep the senses alert (Goleman, 2000). Located in the old emotional brain, the alarm circuit is centered on a series of structures that surround the brainstem and are known as the *limbic system*, so it is the amygdala, located deep in the center of the brain, that plays the main role in emotional emergencies, and which makes us *lose our minds* (Idem). In turn, "the amygdala is the brain's emotional memory bank, a repository of all our moments of triumph and defeat, hope and fear, indignation and frustration" (Goleman, 2000, p.82).

The brain's responses to a crisis still follow the old strategy of suspending complex thinking and triggering automatic responses, generating potentially serious or inconvenient behavior for the person/professional (Goleman, 2000). The amygdala (limbic structure) makes the primary prevail, causing us to react to stimuli, even with behaviors and attitudes that are not socially correct. The amygdala's impulses make emotions prevail over reason (Damásio, 1995; Goleman, 2000). However, Goleman (2000) adds that: "regular, daily practice of a relaxation method seems to reset the amygdala's trigger point to zero, making it less easily provoked" (p.92).

António Damásio (cited by Goleman, 2000) says that the neural centers underlying emotional competence (as opposed to intellectual competence) link the prefrontal region with the emotional centers, concluding in one of his studies that damage to these regions affects the personal and social skills that underlie efficient professional performance, even if intellectual skills remain intact.

These findings confirm that emotion, which emerges from the impulse transmitted between the amygdala and the prefrontal region, is the first phase of a circuit that gives rise to emotion. The prefrontal region houses a set of inhibitory neurons that can veto or cool down impulses from the amygdala (Goleman, 2000). Only then is the neocortex stimulated to transform this emotion - triggering the entire process of reason, depending on the circumstances (Damásio, 1995; Goleman, 2000). As Goleman (2003) points out, based on the studies of LeDoux and Damásio, "(...) the functioning of the amygdala and its interactions with the neocortex are at the heart of emotional intelligence" (p.37).

Goleman, Boyatzis and McKee (2002) introduced the notion of the *open circuit of* the limbic system, referring to the way in which we can be influenced or infected by the emotions of others, and can even change our behaviors and philosophies. They go on to say that many people believe that, from early adulthood onwards, neurological connections atrophy and cannot be replaced, and that adults can no longer change key personal skills. Neurological research has shown just the opposite, as the human brain can create neurological tissue and neurological connections even in adults, which are maintained throughout life (Goleman, Boyatzis and McKee, 2002). Regardless of the stage of life, the neurological circuits that are used the most become stronger, while those that are used infrequently become weaker. Therefore, in order to develop emotional competence and leadership skills later on, there has to be a lot of motivation (Idem).

Damasio (1995), in trying to understand the cognitive and neurological aspects related to reason and emotions, concludes in his studies that "(...) feelings are not as intangible as they have been assumed to be. We may be able to circumscribe them in mental terms, and perhaps we can also find their neurological substrate" (Idem, p.16). This author, during his various observations of brain-injured patients, found associations between reasoning abilities and emotions and feelings, concluding that the body is inextricably integrated and linked to the brain. The researcher goes even further, saying that "If the body and brain interact with each other, the organism they form interacts no less intensely with the environment that surrounds them" (Damásio, 1995, p.106).

Having covered some of the aspects and arguments that have helped to build the concept of emotional intelligence, we will then explain the different EI capacities based on the model presented by Goleman since 1995.

1.4 - THE CAPACITIES OF INTELLIGENCE

EMOTIONAL

First of all, it is important to clarify the concepts of *capacity* and *competence,* since the literature consulted, particularly in English, uses a variety of nomenclature to refer to the same concept. Examples are: *capacity/capacities*; *competence/competencies*; *ability/abilities* and *skill/skills.*

Competence is knowing how to mobilize, integrate and transfer knowledge and skills acquired in training and apply them when necessary in appropriate circumstances, being developed in practice and through knowledge of one's own ability. On the other hand, we understand that **ability** is something that precedes competence. Ability is developed through learning and competence is the way in which people/professionals put it into practice in certain contexts (Berthelof, 1995, Boterf, 1995, Mandoon, 1990, cited by Carvalhal, 1995). According to Howard Gardner (cited by Goleman, 2000), emotional competence is a learned ability, based on EI, which results in extraordinary work performance. Our EI determines our potential to develop practical skills that are based on five capacities: self-awareness, motivation, self-mastery, empathy and relational talent. Thus, our emotional competence shows the extent to which we integrate these skills into our professional competencies (Idem and Ibidem).

For Goleman (2000), Emotional Competence includes emotional and social skills. The author argues that "Emotional competence is a learned ability, based on Emotional Intelligence, that results in extraordinary performance at work. (...) Our emotional competence shows the extent to which we have translated this potential into professional capabilities" (Goleman, 2000, p.33).

Bar-On (cited by Hedlund and Sternberg, 2000, p.147), like Goleman, proposed a model of non-cognitive intelligence which also consists, but in a different way, of five broad areas of specific competencies which each include a set of skills. In short, Bar-On's model (ibid.) consists of:

- Intrapersonal skills: emotional self-awareness, assertiveness, self-actualization, independence and self-regard;
- Interpersonal skills: interpersonal relationships, social responsibility and empathy;
- Adaptability: flexibility, problem-solving and real-life testing;
- Management stress: stress tolerance, impulses and control;
- General mood: happiness and optimism.

Originally, it was Salovey and Mayer (in 1990) who divided Gardner's personal intelligences into four (see p.10) and redefined the abilities of EI (Hedlund and Sternberg, 2000; Salovey, Mayer and Caruso, 2002). Later, Goleman, using the concepts of these authors, presented the concept in an organized and fragmented way in five capacities (Hedlund and Sternberg, 2000). In 1995, Goleman explained the essence of EI abilities (particularly in the educational context) and in 1998 he used the model for work and organizational life, adapting and adding new data to his original model (Goleman, 2000, 2003). Later, in 2002, together with Boyatzis and McKee (2002), he put its importance into perspective in the context of leadership. The author has used different nomenclatures to refer to the same capabilities, depending on the context and approach in which he inserts the concepts. Therefore, in this research, we have adopted the fundamentals of Goleman's original conceptualization (2000, 2003), together with the innovations introduced later by the author for life and work relationships. We have used the original nomenclature for abilities, as we believe that, in essence, there have been no changes in meaning, but only slight adaptations according to the context in which they are applied. We chose not to isolate the models because we believe that one complements the other, and we also wanted to give a perspective not only on the importance of emotional skills in the workplace, but also on the development and education of these skills.

Table 1 shows an adaptation of the relationship between the five major EI competencies and the twenty-five emotional dimensions.

Personal competence
These skills determine how we manage ourselves
Self-awareness
(Knowing our inner states, preferences, resources and intuitions)
Emotional self-awareness: recognizing your own emotions and their effects **Self-evaluation requires:** knowing your own strengths and limitations **Self-confidence:** confidence in one's abilities and self-worth
Emotion management
(Managing one's own internal states, impulses and resources)
Self-mastery: managing negative emotions and impulses **Inspiring trust:** maintaining standards of honesty and integrity **Being conscientious:** taking responsibility for personal performance **Adaptability:** flexibility in dealing with change **Innovation:** feeling comfortable and open to new ideas, approaches and information
Automotive
(Emotional tendencies that guide or facilitate the achievement of goals)
Will to succeed: striving to improve or reach a standard of excellence **Commitment:** aligning with the objectives of the group or organization **Initiative:** being prepared to seize opportunities **Optimism:** persistence in pursuing goals despite obstacles and setbacks
Social Competence
These skills determine how we deal with relationships.
Empathy
(Awareness of the feelings, needs and concerns of others)
Understanding others: being aware of the feelings and perspectives of others and taking an active interest in their concerns. **Developing others:** being aware of the development needs of others and strengthening their capacities **Service orientation:** anticipating, recognizing and meeting customer needs **Enhancing diversity:** cultivating opportunities with different types of people **Political awareness:** reading the emotional currents and power relations of a group
Group relationship management
(Ability to induce favorable responses in others)
Influence: using effective persuasion tactics **Communication:** listening openly and sending convincing messages **Conflict management:** negotiating and resolving disagreements **Leadership:** inspiring and guiding groups and people **Catalyst for change:** initiating and managing change **Creating bonds:** nurturing instrumental relationships **Collaboration and cooperation:** working with others towards common goals **Team skills:** creating group synergies in pursuit of collective goals

Chart 1 - Emotional competence model, adapted from Goleman (2000; 2003)
These skills are divided into two main areas: personal skills, which determine how we manage ourselves, and social skills, which refer to how we deal with relationships (Goleman, 2000, 2003). Thus, according to this conceptual model, Emotional Intelligence is based on five major abilities: self-awareness, managing emotions, self-motivation, empathy and managing relationships in groups.

1.4.1 - Self-awareness

From this perspective, self-awareness is the way we identify our own emotions while they are happening. For the author, this is the basis of EI, which translates into self-knowledge, the result of analyzing oneself, one's own life, how one behaves and how one wishes to behave (Goleman, 2000).

Here, the author emphasizes the role of self-awareness, i.e. the importance of becoming aware of the negative emotions in our lives (anxiety, aggression and melancholy), as the best way to adapt to the situation we are facing. Knowing and recognizing what we feel through a real self-assessment of our own emotions/feelings is something that gives us self-confidence and guides us when making a decision (Goleman, 2003).

People who don't understand their feelings are unconsciously surrendering to them. People who know and interpret their feelings guide their lives in a more stable and productive way (Goleman, 2003). In the words of this researcher: "People who have greater certainty about their feelings govern their lives better, having a more secure sense of what they really feel about the decisions they have to make, from who to marry to what job to take." (Goleman, 2003, p. 63).

1.4.2 - Being a manager of your emogoes

The ability to manage one's own emotions refers to how we manage the emotions we may face. It shows that self-knowledge aims to provide self-encounter, seeking the constant improvement of oneself as a person through self-control, controlling impulses/emotions in a healthy way and thinking before acting, in order to achieve happiness in the contexts in which one is inserted (Goleman, 2000). Managing emotions emerges from self-knowledge and results in self-regulation so that, instead of hindering, they facilitate the task at hand. It is also a way of "dealing with feelings in an appropriate way (...)" (Goleman, 2003, p.63).

Negotiating with ourselves in order to achieve personal stability is the starting point for a correct connection between the world and the people around us, so that, at certain times, managing our emotions implies the right way to take out our anger or bad mood on the right person (Goleman, 2003). The author also says that people who possess this quality to a high degree "recover much more quickly from the falls that life forces us to take" (p.63).

1.4.3 - Staying Motivated

Self-motivation is the way we use our energy from a constructive and projective perspective. Discovering self-motivation means finding the reasons that drive us to work for reasons that go beyond money or social prominence. A motivated person or professional is someone who puts persistence and reason into their goals (Goleman, 2000). The same author reminds us that in order to take initiatives and be highly efficient in the face of setbacks and frustrations, we need to use our deepest preferences, which allow us to move towards our goals (Goleman, 2003).

The ability to self-motivate is understood as a way of remaining optimistic in the face of problems or unpleasant situations. According to Goleman (2003, p.63), "People who possess this ability tend to be more highly productive and effective in everything they do".

1.4.4 - Perceiving and interpreting the emotions of others

Like the previous abilities, it can be called different things. Thus, the ability to *recognize the emotions of others* is often referred to as empathy. It encompasses verbal and non-verbal expression and the way we perceive and interpret the emotions of others, having a sense of what people feel, being able to adopt their perspective and cultivating bonds and attunement with other people (Goleman, 2003).

The EI competencies are linked to each other and apply to both the individual and the group. The fact that individuals in a group empathize with each other leads the group to create and develop positive norms for managing the group's relationships with the outside world (Goleman, Boyatzis and McKee, 2002). According to these authors, at the level of social awareness, empathy is the basis on which the team builds relationships with the rest of the organization (Idem).

As Goleman (2000) points out, empathy is fundamental to success in interpersonal relationships. It is the ability to understand the emotions of others in accordance with their emotional responses. In teamwork, this ability takes on its full significance in promoting and developing an organizational climate conducive to good practice. This ability is considered a fundamental quality for professionals in the fields of care, teaching, sales and management (Goleman, 2003).

1.4.5 - Managing relationships in groups

The ability to manage relationships in groups is also known as group emotion management (Goleman, 2000). In the modern world, it is essential to develop effective relationships in a group or team. Communication, leadership and teamwork skills are key to success in a competitive workplace (Goleman, 2000). Managing relationships in groups is a social skill that consists of knowing how to read the situations of a group (social, family, professional) well, in order to have the ability to manage relationships within a group - formal or informal (Goleman, 2003). It means being able to harmoniously relate your skills to persuade, lead, negotiate, work as part of a team and resolve conflicts efficiently (Idem).

Assertiveness training is essential for establishing effective relationships (pedagogical, therapeutic, personal and professional), in order to deal well with the emotional reactions of others and when faced with stressful emotional situations. According to Goleman (2003, p.64), "It is these skills that underlie popularity, leadership and interpersonal effectiveness". It could be said that Goleman is an adherent of the notion that more emotionally competent people have a more positive relationship with themselves and others than those who suffer from some level of *emotional illiteracy* (Branco, 2004b; Goleman, 2003).

With this background, we can conclude that although each author and researcher has their own conception of EI, each of them develops it based on their experiences, giving rise to theories with slight differences, but which together complement and do not contradict each other. Daniel Goleman, as well as being the most popular, is, in our opinion, the most practical and objective author in what he develops, and can serve as a basic model for applying the concept to the professional nursing group, as well as providing a foundation for research in this area.

Chapter 2

2 - A MEASURING INSTRUMENT

If we want to know what people think, feel and believe, the most direct way of obtaining information is to ask them, so interview and survey techniques are the means to use (Polit and Hungler, 1995). In this chapter, we will look at the measuring instrument adopted, the procedures for adapting it and the variables it encompasses.

Considering that quantitative methodology is appropriate for this type of study, there is a need for measuring instruments. In choosing the instrument that could best address this issue, reference was made to the target population and the reality to be studied.

When we chose the measuring instrument in question - a questionnaire - we took into account what these authors say about data collection by this means (Polit and Hungler, 1995):

- "The questions need to be in a sequence, in a psychologically meaningful order and in a way that encourages collaboration and frankness." (p. 68);
- "Questionnaires offer the possibility of total anonymity, which can be fundamental in obtaining information about socially unacceptable behavior." (p.170);
- "The absence of an interviewer ensures that there is no bias in the answers, which reflect the respondent's reaction to the interviewer and not the questions themselves." (p.170).

But these are not just advantages. Several authors, such as Ghiglione and Matalon (2001) and Quivy and Campenhoudt (1998), mention some limitations and disadvantages of the questionnaire, such as the fact that it can be expensive, that the answers are superficial and that it involves individualizing the respondents. However, according to Ghiglione and Matalon (2001), the questionnaire is a standardized instrument, both in the wording of the questions and in their order, with the aim of guaranteeing the comparability of responses from all individuals, estimating absolute and relative quantities, describing a population or verifying hypotheses. This last argument led us to opt for this type of instrument. Having opted for the questionnaire format for data collection, we were faced with another question: *Which scale or test to adopt, given the various existing ones (each with its own specificity)?*

Various tests have already been developed with the aim of testing the personal qualities that most result in EI and improve performance. Based on the theories of authors such as Martin Seligman, Bar-On, Goleman, Boyatzis, Salovey and Mayer, among others, these tests have been used on various groups, including: recruits, executives/leaders, athletes, students and patients (Cherniss, 2000).

Pérez González (2004), a professor at the Faculty of Education, after more than 10 years of research into emotional intelligence (EI), has found a wide variety of instruments to measure it, spread across several countries. Even so, only a few of them have reliable and valid psychometric characteristics. According to this author, EI researchers should be able to distinguish between at least three types of measures: a) Maximum performance tests (or ability tests that measure EI abilities); b) Self-report questionnaires (or performance tests that measure specific EI characteristics); and c) 360-degree assessments or other informative questionnaires (which measure trends in EI characteristics or emotional competence, when the items use behavioral indicators). These three types of measures use three different measurement criteria: a) Objective; b) Subjective; and c) Intra-subjective, respectively.

Although the definition and validation of a new construct depends on the instruments used to measure it, to date there are only a few detailed and important critical studies that review the multiple measures of EI and related constructs (Schutte and Malouff, 1999; Ciarrochi et al., 2001, Mathews et al., 2002, MacCann et al., in press, Cit by Pérez González, 2004).

In a very practical way, Pérez González (2004) presents a poster of his own, which consists of a table classifying the best-known EI measurements in chronological order, as well as a short description of their main technical characteristics and psychometric features. With this work, the author has essentially tried to synthesize the diverse information available on EI assessment instruments. It summarizes the main (and perhaps most relevant) instruments studied in relation to this scientific field in recent years. However, some of these instruments have been popularized through non-scientific literature (popular literature on EI) in which, for the most part, an amalgam of constructs is used.

Given the wide range of existing instruments, the choice and accessibility were not easy, so several could be adapted to our model. However, most of them are foreign and have *limitations* in terms of use and access. These instruments are: time-consuming to fill in, made in a different cultural context (foreigners), requiring iraducao. expensive to purchase. and some of the authors require that they process the data themselves. Gasquet (2000) also points out that the social and cultural differences between developed countries, both in terms of the functioning of health systems and collective representations of health, do not allow for the direct transposition (by simple translation) of measurement and evaluation instruments. In view of these and other constraints, we decided to adopt an EI scale that had already been properly constructed in Portuguese and to assess it against the reality of clinical nursing practice.

In Portugal, we found two EI measurement instruments created in Portugal that could be adapted to the characteristics of our population. The first, by Rego and Fernandes (in press), was validated in 2003 on a sample of 77 professors and non-teaching staff from the University of Aveiro, 177 students and 85 employees from a large industrial company in central Portugal. The second was created and validated in 1999 by Branco. The fact that these scales are Portuguese immediately struck us as an advantage, as this avoided *cultural* problems.

We then had to decide between the two, and opted for the latter for the reasons explained below:

- Augusta Veiga Branco is a Nurse and Professor of Nursing at the Escola Superior de Saúde de Braganga, and her scientific interests include the study of EI. She has published several papers in this area. She invests in her academic development by combining education with EI, and has a PhD in Educational Sciences;
- The scale emerged from her Master's dissertation with the aim of characterizing and identifying behaviour and attitudes in emotional situations in a sample of 250 school teachers.

  - public and private universities in the district of Braganga (Branco, 2004b);
- He later used the Self-motivation sub-scale in a study of 250 nursing students from public and private higher education in the district of Braganga (Branco, 2004a);
- In her doctoral thesis, the author used the same scale on a sample of 464 primary

and secondary school teachers from the district of Braganga (Branco, 2005);

- The accessibility and previous validations gave us the security of use;
- The author made herself available to accompany the process of adapting the scale to the new population by joining the group of experts, with the aim of not distorting the original matrix of the instrument.

The author's *background* combined with the fact that her basic training is in nursing, as well as the studies she has already carried out using and testing the scale, which has proved to be valid and reliable, are reasons that justify our choice. We believe that when the questions/items of the questionnaire, based on Daniel Goleman's EI model, were formulated, the author could not detach herself from her professional training and experience in nursing. When we read her questionnaire in its original version, we were able to fit each item perfectly into the professional context of nursing. Also, according to the author's reports during the formal interviews, this instrument is designed, in its basic conception, for people in general and not for any particular profile of person/professional. What it does need is an adjustment to the framing of some of the items in order to direct the questions and contextualize situations that apply to the new population - nurses.

2.1 - EVB-CIE: ORIGINAL VERSA

In 1999, Veiga Branco used the conceptualization (descriptions and concepts) of Goleman's EI to construct the set of statements and items for his scale. In terms of the operationalization of the concepts, each of the abilities was used as conceptual units, translating them into statements and expressions, maintaining the meaning that Goleman attributed to them in each of the five domains, in order to construct an instrument of closed questions to be able to test the teacher's emotional competence (Branco, 2004b). From a practical point of view, **five sub-scales** were constructed rather than a single scale. The author justifies this as follows:

"From the point of view of the concepts and the instruments that can measure them, it is considered that it is not possible to treat the five capacities as a whole, not only because the author himself elaborated and presented the concept of *Emotional Intelligence* fragmented into five different domains, but also and above all, because as a whole they assess five different dimensions of the subject's psychic system." (Branco, 2004b, p.86).

In relation to this option, Salovey, Mayer and Caruso (2002) also point out that, although there is sometimes empirical utility in considering emotional intelligence as a unitary construct, the model they built can also be divided into four sets of abilities.

Adopting Goleman's model (2000, 2003), each of the EI capacities measures different phenomena, because they belong to different levels, although they can sometimes manifest themselves in similar attitudes or behaviors, indicating as a whole a configuration of the EI of the sample to which the instrument is applied. In constructing the scale, the author based herself on some assumptions, which we will now mention (Branco, 2004b):

- EI is a fragmented construct and is operationalized in five capacities, respecting Goleman's model;
- Each ability is a construct, which has been operationalized by identifying the behaviours, feelings and attitudes that characterize it. These form a set of five sub-scales;
- To identify these behaviors, feelings and attitudes, Goleman's descriptions and expressions were used, maintaining the meaning that the author attributed to them;
- It is hoped that the content of the statements/items will somehow translate what the

subjects feel. If the respondents, by marking the answers, understand that the contents make sense from their point of view of the emotions they experience, then this means that they are corroborating the sense and meaning of the theoretical assumptions used to construct the instrument;

- The behaviors, feelings and attitudes are decoded into statements (items) which correspond to a Likert-type scale - of temporal frequency - for the respondents to mark how often they experience the emotional phenomena or hypothetical situations described;
- Respondents are asked to mentally place themselves in a given hypothetical situation and to indicate (in their own perception) how often these attitudes or behaviors occur to them;
- The procedure described above is repeated for each of the five sub-scales, resulting in a data collection scale that groups together five different scales.

After carrying out the respective operationalization, the author tested the instrument on a sample of teachers to check whether these abilities or domains were as Goleman conceptualizes them. In this study, the author obtained 18 factors, divided into five sub-scales, with Cronbach's alphas starting at 0.54 - in the factors, and higher than 0.68 in the sub-scales (Branco, 1999). The global scale, originally organized and created to measure teachers' EI capacities, was later called: Veiga Branco Scale of Emotional Intelligence Capacities (EVB-CIE). Thus, and respecting the principles described above, the original scale has a total of 85 items, divided into five sub-scales (Idem):

1. Capacity for **Self-Awareness** (20 items);
2. **Emotion Management** Capacity (18 items);
3. **Automotive** capacity (21 items);
4. **Empathy** Capacity (12 items);
5. **Group Relationship Management** Capacity (14 items).

2.2 - ADAPTED TO THE NURSING POPULATION

After choosing the scale, there was a need to refine and adapt it since the context in which the questions were presented was not suitable for the population of nurses. So, after receiving the author's permission, we made the necessary adaptations to apply the questionnaire to the *new population, taking* care not to change the *meaning of* the contexts in which the items are inserted. To do this, we brought together a group of experts and carried out a pre-test, as explained below.

2.2.1 - Group of experts

As suggested by Fortin (1999), the questionnaire was submitted to expert analysis in order to verify its content validity and to ensure that this measuring instrument is representative of the domain to be assessed. The group was made up of six experts who agreed to take part and who met at least one of the following inclusion criteria:

- Knowledge of the area under study (IE and people management);
- Knowledge of the scale that made up the questionnaire (author's own);
- Knowledge of nursing, particularly in relation to work contexts and the technical language used by nurses.

Discussions about the changes to be made took place in March and April. During these moments of sharing, changes emerged in the contextualization of the scale and some of the questions in the characterization of the sample in order to direct it towards nursing practice. Examples include:

- "Imagine a professional activity **(wound care, bladder catheterization, teaching the patient/family, etc.)**. During the activity, I usually feel that: (...)", instead of "Imagine a professional activity **(teaching session, bibliographical research, attending to students, etc.)**. During the activity, I usually feel that: (...)";
- "On average, how many **hours do you work per week (at this and another institution)**?", instead of "On average, how many **classes do you teach per week**?".

It was also decided to include an open-ended item in each set of expressions. This gives the respondent the opportunity to put forward a behavior or attitude that is not included in the original items, and is also located on the seven-point Likert scale. The item is called *other* and is optional, as explained in the procedure for filling in the questionnaire.

Another point proposed by the group of experts was to ask the nurses surveyed to put the questionnaire in a sealed envelope after completing it, thus guaranteeing the privacy of the participants in the study. This was necessary because the data collection strategy adopted involved the participation of the head nurses of each service in the distribution and collection of the questionnaires.

2.2.2 - Pre-Test

After the discussion and the suggested changes/adaptations in the expert group, we also thought it appropriate to carry out a pre-test before applying the questionnaire. Our aim was to determine whether the questionnaire was written clearly and without bias, whether it asked for the type of information required and whether the layout allowed it to be filled in correctly. We also wanted to identify any possible flaws in the instrument and to find out the average time taken to complete the questionnaire, bearing in mind that nurses are professionals who work shifts and often in several workplaces, so it is not always easy to obtain their cooperation and availability.

The pre-test was administered to a total of 20 nurses - 11 teachers from the former Sao Joao School of Nursing and nine nurses from a hospital. The questionnaires were handed out on May 3, 2004 and collected within a week. Each nurse was asked to make any changes they considered necessary, but always without detracting from the original number and content of the items.

After analyzing the comments made on the questionnaire, it was decided to accept some of the suggested changes:

- Refining the structural aspect to make it easier to fill in (e.g. including the Likert scale legend on all sheets);
- Change the explanation of the filling procedure to make it clearer;
- Include some variables in the characterization of the sample, such as - *immigrant*

(with their nationality), *number of dependents and weekly working hours*.

It should be noted that, with regard to the content of the scale (adapted for data collection), the same items as the original scale were kept. The subjects involved in the pre-test also confirmed the suggestions made by the group of experts.

2.2.3 - Adapted version

In order to characterize the population under study, test the research questions posed and verify the relationships between some of the variables chosen, we divided the questionnaire into two parts. The first contains essential questions for characterizing the sample, which focus on personal characteristics and also on the importance attributed to relationships and dialogues in the respondents' professional context. The second part aims to find out each nurse's personal perception of their level of ability in each of the EI skills, using the EVB-CIE. The latter consists of a total of 85 statements/expressions, organized into five distinct groups - corresponding to the five EI skills - where hypothetical situations appear, with the aim of inducing the respondent to identify with them. Each of the situations corresponds to one or more sets of expressions, and each of these expressions corresponds to a time-frequency scale, which aims to identify the frequency with which the attitudes or behaviors expressed are experienced by the respondents.

Each of the expressions is answered using a Likert scale, which corresponds to the time frequency in which each situation occurs, varying on a *continuum* between *Never* and *Always*. Thus, the values can be: 1 - never, 2 - rarely, 3 - infrequently, 4 - usually, 5 - frequently, 6 - very frequently and 7 - always. For each set of expressions, respondents also have the option of giving an open-ended answer on the *other* item.

For the whole scale, the higher the value given (on the Likert scale), the greater the agreement with the statement and the EI capacity analyzed. The way we found to collect data, with closed questions followed by Likert-type scales (1-7), has the advantage of being easier to answer and can be subjected to more rigorous statistical treatments. We have therefore prepared the variables of the instrument to be applied to a sample of nurses from an EPE Hospital, in the hope that the results will reveal the configurations of each of the EI capacities and of EI as a whole.

2.2.4 - The variables involved

In correlational studies, the variables are essentially related to the dimensions of the behaviors being assessed or the traits being assessed (Almeida and Freire, 2000). In this adaptation we have the following variables: those characterizing the sample and those making up the factors (after finding the respective factor solutions), EI abilities and emotional intelligence (as a whole).

In part I of the questionnaire, the variables that characterize the sample in socio-demographic terms are: *Age, Gender, Immigrant, Number of dependents, Academic qualifications, Postgraduate training* and *Other specific training*. We considered including the *Immigrant* variable because we realized that, in the institution where we collected the data, there was a significant percentage of Spanish nurses who had moved from their country specifically to work. These nurses have a different academic background and culture to the Portuguese, which could mean differences in their self-perception of their EI skills. As for the professional level variables, we added: *Length of service; Contractual relationship; Professional category; Weekly working hours; Service; Liking the workplace; Their ideas are listened to and put into practice; Considering adequate working conditions* and *Feeling fulfilled as a nurse.*

We also considered other variables that we felt were relevant to relate to EI skills, noting that some of them were used (measured by teachers) in Augusta Veiga Branco's original questionnaire. These are Do you *consider your interpersonal relationships with patients to be important for the success of the care you provide?*; Do *you consider your emotional stability to be important in your interpersonal relationships with others (patients, multidisciplinary team, bosses, etc.)?*; *Do you consider your relationships with people (family or social) to be important for your emotional stability?*; *Throughout your experience as a nurse, do you consider that you have experienced the care process with levels of success?*; and *Nowadays, being a nurse is...?* In these questions, the participant had the option of answering on a five-point Likert scale. In the first three, 1 (one) corresponds to *unimportant* and 5 (five) to *very important*. In the fourth question, 1 (one) corresponds to *very low* and 5 (five) to *very high*. In the last question, 1 (one) means *not at all rewarding and 5 (*five) means *very rewarding*. In the last items mentioned, we sought to obtain data on satisfaction with their work. We didn't choose to use job satisfaction scales from the literature, as we felt they didn't fit in with the objectives of the study.

Part I also includes the operationalization of the *Service* variable, which was treated in a special way. To do this, we assumed that, depending on the characteristics of the service in which nurses work, nurses establish different interpersonal relationships, both with users and their families, and with other professionals. These relationships can be distinguished in terms of: - the length of contact that exists for the therapeutic relationship (which implies differences in the relationship and involvement with the user/citizen); - the existence or not of verbal communication with the user; and - the differences related to the specific aims and objectives of the operation of each service.

During the data collection period of the study, we had the opportunity to get to know the existing services better, as well as the differences in interaction established within the multi-professional teams and between the nurses and the users of each unit. This way, and based on the *Service* variable, we created a new variable called *Type of Service* - related to the type and duration of the relationship established with the user. It was defined as a dichotomous variable, with two secondary groups. One group, called *Acute*, includes services where nurses establish therapeutic relationships in shorter periods of time or where verbal communication is often impossible or reduced (due to the clinical condition of the patients). In the opposite group, *chronic* care, we have included services where the therapeutic relationships established are, as a rule, longer-lasting (the case of inpatient care) and the relationship established between the agents involved in the care is more in-depth and stronger, in terms of the development of interpersonal relationships with the users.

Based on these principles and our personal and professional perception, we believe that, depending on the characteristics of the type of service in which nurses work, they may develop different EI skills. Thus, in the *Type of Service* variable, we included in the group - *Acute* - nurses belonging to the following services: Emergency, Intermediate Care Unit, Multipurpose Intensive Care Unit, Operating Room and Birth Center. *In* the *Chronic* group, we include nurses working in the following services: Private Rooms (Otorhinolaryngology, Ophthalmology and Urology), General and Plastic Surgery, Orthopedics, Obstetrics and

Gynecology, General Medicine, Medical Oncology, Pediatrics and Neonatology. The name of the groups will not be the one that best reflects their content, but it will certainly serve to verify whether or not there are differences between them and the capabilities of the EI.

Assuming that the items on the EVB-CIE, adapted for nurses, reflect the five abilities outlined by Goleman in 1995, and that these are correlated with nurses' EI, we were able to proceed with a study to find out nurses' profiles in relation to each of these abilities and their overall EI.

PART II

FROM THEORY TO
RESEARCH RESULTS

This part of the book presents the first research in Portugal into the emotional intelligence of nurses. The study was carried out as part of the Master's Degree in Public Management, specializing in People Management, presented to the Autonomous Section of Social, Legal and Political Sciences at the University of Aveiro.

The methodological choices that led to the study will be discussed, with reference to: the contextualization and justification; the data collection procedures; the statistical treatment of the data and, finally, the presentation of the main results of the research.

Chapter 3

3 - THE CONTEXT OF THE STUDY

The dissatisfaction of users and professionals is mentioned as one of the problems in the National Health Service (Portugal. Ministério da Saúde, 1997). We believe that much of the dissatisfaction of users and professionals themselves is due to the fact that they don't make the most of their emotional capacities in order to manage their professional and personal lives in the most effective way. As nurses are the largest group of health professionals working in multi-professional teams, there is a constant need to manage relationships with patients and other team members.

In the conclusions of a study conducted by Branco (2004b) on the emotional intelligence (EI) of teachers in Polytechnic Higher Education in the district of Bragança, the author suggests that: "It would be entirely pertinent to repeat all the assumptions and methodological processes, in this or other populations, in this or other areas of work, as long as emotional competence was considered important" (p.114). Considering this proposal to be valid for the professional nursing group, we accepted the challenge of studying the reality of EI skills in a sample of nurses from a hospital organization.

PURPOSE AND OBJECTIVES

Based on the contextualization of this research, and believing that the

Since EI is important in the professional context of nurses, we aim to contribute to improving human resource management, for the purposes of organizing and training nurses. Knowing the purpose of the study, we also identified the following objectives:

- To validate a measuring instrument capable of measuring nurses' EI skills;

- To characterize the profile of each of the EI capacities of the nurses studied, based on their personal self-perception, ultimately revealing a global configuration of their EI;
- To identify some variables that influence nurses' EI;
- Check how EI capabilities correlate with each other and with global EI;
- Recognize the predictive variables of EI.

RESEARCH QUESTIONS

Assuming the real importance of knowing nurses' EI skills for the training and management of this professional group, we will focus all our research on these skills. Based on the questions that have arisen throughout the research and theoretical foundation, we have now defined four research questions, conceptually looking for something to guide us throughout the execution of the study design, fulfilling the objectives and purpose of this work.

We can then pose the following research questions:

Question 1: What is the potential of the Veiga Branco Emotional Intelligence Capacities Scale to measure nurses' EI capacities?

Question 2: What configuration does the population of nurses studied have with regard to EI capabilities?

Question 3: What variables influence nurses' abilities and EI?

Question 4: Could knowledge of EI capabilities be a contribution to the management and training of this professional group?

At the end of the study, we hope to be able to answer the questions that have now been raised, allowing us to analyze and understand the characteristics of nurses' EI in the light of Goleman's theoretical model and through the Veiga Branco Scale of Emotional Intelligence Capacities.

TYPE OF STUDY

This point refers to the description of the structure used, based on the central questions of the research, whether it aims to describe variables or groups of subjects, explore or examine relationships between variables or even verify hypotheses of causality (Fortin, 2000).

We chose to carry out an exploratory study, given the scarcity of studies carried out and the fact that we were studying EI in a population of nurses in Portugal for the first time. We can also say that, as well as being exploratory, this is a descriptive and correlational study. According to Fortin (2000), descriptive studies are exploratory studies that stem from the fact that the researcher does not necessarily have a set of well-developed assumptions to formulate hypotheses, but provides a description of the data in the form of words, numbers or descriptive statements of relationships between variables. The author adds that this type of study "consists of describing a phenomenon or concept relating to a population, in order to establish the characteristics of this population or a sample of it" (Fortin, 2000, p.163). However, in this study, we do not intend to take an explanatory approach to the situational and institutional reality, but only to provide clues that will allow us to consider future decisions with a view to the management and training of nurses. Issues such as recruitment, selection, evaluation, performance improvement, teamwork and emotional education are aspects to which we hope to contribute.

Also, as in the study by Branco (1999), we wanted to find out whether a set of constructs (sub-scales that make up the global scale) can reveal a perceived reality, whether there is a correlation between these constructs, and whether there are relationships between these constructs/abilities and emotional intelligence.

As far as the research method is concerned, the approach used to obtain information and describe a phenomenon can be qualitative or quantitative. Thus, we will use the quantitative research paradigm, which consists of "manipulating numerical data, using statistical procedures, in order to describe phenomena or assess the magnitude and reliability of relationships between them" (Polit and Hungler, 1995, p.358-359).

POPULATION AND SAMPLE

Polit and Hungler (1995, p.143) define a population as "any aggregation of cases that meet a chosen set of criteria". Fortin (2000, p.373) also defines a population as "all the subjects or other elements of a well-defined group which share one or more similar characteristics and on which the research is based". Taking these definitions as a starting point, it was established that the population of this study is made up of all nurses with a contractual relationship to the EPE Hospital where the study was carried out, i.e. all nurses who belong to the public sector, with a fixed-term contract (CTC) or with an open-ended contract (permanent). In this way, we wanted to include all nurses who had an *identity* with the aforementioned institution and who were integrated into the organizational dynamic. We excluded what are known as casual *nurses* and those hired to replace vacations, because they do not have a continuous collaboration with the hospital in question.

With regard to the sample, it is considered to be the process of selecting a part of the population to represent its totality (Polit and Hungler, 1995). Lortin (2000, p.363) also adds that "it is the set of operations that consists of choosing a group of subjects or any other representative element of the population studied". To calculate the minimum sample size, we multiplied the number of items in the largest sub-scale, out of the five that make up the data collection instrument used, by seven (the maximum value of the Likert scale used for each answer), ignoring the *answer-other* items. In this way, the instrument was validated sub-scale by sub-scale. Furthermore, treating each ability/sub-scale independently does not distort the concept of EI, as it respects the theoretical model advocated by Goleman and the instrument's own validation methodology used by Branco in 1999.

For convenience, we chose to study the total population of the nurses mentioned, and there was no need to use sampling techniques. This was due to the fact that the population was known, finite, not very large and could be studied in its entirety, consisting of 314 nurses, according to the data provided (on June 9, 2004) by the Nurse Director of the hospital where this study was carried out.

From the outset, we can consider the overall receptiveness of nurses to the study to be very satisfactory. A total of 214 nurses answered the questionnaire, which corresponds to an adherence rate of 68.2%. It is clear that the number of respondents is not equal to the number of people who make up the population, so our sample consists of the 214 nurses who answered the questionnaire. According to Fortin (1999), the sample, being a subset of the population under study, is representative of the target population. It is representative not only of the variables under study, but also of the socio-professional characteristics themselves (Fortin, 1999, 2000; Polit and Hungler, 1995). Once we know the sample, we can recall that our object of study was defined as the emotional intelligence skills of nurses in a hospital setting.

3.1 - THE PHASES

The study began with a review of the literature, with the object of study being the emotional intelligence skills of nurses in the hospital context. From this bibliographical research, with an emphasis on Daniel Goleman's model of EI, emerged concerns and questions that could be investigated, which gave rise to the study itself.

Having defined the study population and the sample to be studied, it is now important to show the stages involved in carrying out the study. We will begin by describing the data collection instrument, as well as the procedures for adapting it to the population under analysis. At the same time, we will present the variables under study - which emerged from the bibliographical research of previous studies and from our own empirical experience.

Once the data collection instrument has been determined, the explanations explaining how the data was collected follow. Once the data has been collected, the data is statistically processed and the results obtained from the sample emerge - both in terms of socio-professional characteristics and the EI skills of the nurses under study.

With the new data obtained, it will be possible to compare it with the theoretical concepts of various authors (particularly Goleman) and with the results found in other studies already carried out in the area. At the end of this research, it will be possible to highlight the main conclusions of the study, as well as the possible contributions that the study could make to the various levels of nursing training and activity.

3.2 - THE METHOD

The data was collected in an EPE Hospital, as this gave us greater guarantees of obtaining a significant and diverse sample of nurses - in terms of the health services provided. The data collection instrument (questionnaire) was distributed and collected between June 22 and August 27, 2004. Each nurse was asked to answer all the questions, as explained in the completion procedure. At the end of completing the questionnaire, they were asked to seal it in an envelope provided.

Once the data has been collected, we move on to processing the information obtained. This chapter will describe the operations carried out to validate the instrument used on the population of nurses studied, the statistical analysis of the variables, the correlational study and the analysis of the predictive variables of emotional intelligence.

At the beginning of this study, we set out to carry out an exploratory, descriptive and correlational study, with the aim of validating the Veiga Branco Scale of Emotional Intelligence Capacities and finding out about the emotional intelligence (EI) capacities of the nurses studied. Since there is already a validation and fidelity study on a sample of teachers, using the same scale, we intend to develop the research in order to obtain some reference data for future studies and to compare the results of our sample with existing studies.

Once the data had been collected, it was entered into a database and then processed using the statistical data analysis program SPSS (Statistical Package for Social Sciences) version 12.0. According to Polit and Hungler (1995, p.227), "Without the help of statistics, the quantitative data collected in a research project is little more than a chaotic mass of numbers. Statistical procedures enable the researcher to reduce, summarize, organize, evaluate, interpret and communicate numerical information". To this end, we selected different statistical procedures, depending on the objectives to be achieved.

In order to get to know the sample better through the first part of the questionnaire, descriptive analysis was used, with absolute and relative frequency values, by single variable or, when considered relevant, by crossing variables (using the SPSS *Crosstabs* command).

In the second part of the questionnaire - the Veiga Branco Scale of EI Capabilities - where each sub-scale measures a capability, revealing as a whole the configuration of the sample's EI through the answers obtained, principal component analysis was carried out with Varimax orthogonal rotation. Factor analysis was extended to each of the five sub-scales (capabilities), independently, with a view to validating the constructs in a new population.

To construct the factors, we used the previous validation with teachers (Branco, 2004b), without distorting the way in which this sample groups them, and taking into account the verification of the variance values. According to Pestana and Gageiro (2003), exploratory factorial analysis was essentially carried out, but also as a confirmatory technique. In some cases, the desired number of factors to be retained was chosen in advance, based on theory and, in particular, on Branco's previous validation, in order to understand whether or not the factorial solution was similar to that of the teachers. Factor analysis made it possible to verify the interrelationships between the variables by grouping them into factors and assigning a name to each of these groupings (Polit and Hungler, 1997).

To name the factors, we used the nomenclature used by Branco, in the validation with teachers, when they included the same items. It was only changed when the emerging factors varied in at least one item. The classification of these factors was essentially a process of identifying theoretical constructs, making it possible to organize the way subjects interpret the situations indicated, indicating which are related and which are not. It also made it possible to assess the validity of the variables included in each factor, indicating the extent to which they refer to the same concepts, through the correlation between them (Pestana and Gageiro, 2003).

The inclusion and exclusion criteria for the items to be included in each factor,

we took into account:

- Selection of items with saturation greater than 0.30;
- Saturation in more than one factor was included in the factor in which the saturation value was highest (unless its descriptive interpretation did not justify it);
- Items with only negative saturations were recoded and their content analyzed;
- For items with positive saturation in one factor and negative saturation in another, we analyzed their descriptive power, checking in which factor the item made the most sense (taking into account its theoretical basis).

After this analysis, we proceeded to describe the results obtained using the *Reliability Analysis*

- *Scale (Alpha)* statistical procedure, determining the *Cronbach's alpha* coefficient (internal consistency) for each factor and sub-scale, with the aim of verifying the reliability of the *scale*.

each sub-scale and the overall scale. In each of these analyses, factors with an eigenvalue greater than 1.0 (one) and a minimum internal validity expression of 0.50 were considered.

The sample's response values were also analyzed, both in relation to the factors extracted by the previous analysis, and in relation to each of the EI abilities and overall emotional intelligence. To obtain the distribution of the sample for each variable, we determined the minimum and maximum scores, the average of the actual sums obtained for each of the variables in question, and the respective standard deviation, which determined the distribution of the sample: X ± 1DP. In order to facilitate the analysis of the results, we corresponded the distribution of responses for each factor and ability to the values 1 (one) and 7 (seven) on the Likert scale, which correspond (respectively) to: *never, rarely, infrequently, usually, frequently, very frequently* and *always*. This correspondence was made possible by calculating the weighted average, obtained by dividing the value of the average by the number of items in each factor, ability and overall EI.

In order to confirm the results of the distribution with the widest range of responses, we used percentile tables (associated with whisker graphs) which allowed us to find the distribution of all the responses in the sample (Min-Max) and also where 50% of the responses were. According to Pestana and Gageiro (2003, p.84), "The difference between percentiles or deciles associated with the minimum and maximum values of the data gives an idea of the dispersion or concentration of the data".

We used measures of central tendency (mean and standard deviation) to describe the distribution of responses in the various EI factors and skills, even though the distribution was not normal for all of our factors and for four of our skills. We used these measures, based on the central limit theory, because the mean in most situations is very close to the median, which is almost always between the minimum and maximum value for the mean in a 95% confidence interval (Marroco, 2003).

Statistical tests were also applied to see if there were any statistically significant differences between some of the variables that characterized the sample and the factors, skills and Emotional Intelligence. In choosing these variables, we relied on the literature and the fact that they had already been used in a previous study with the same scale (in teachers). The following variables were selected: **Gender, Age** (< 40 years >), **Immigrant, Academic qualifications, Type of service** and **Postgraduate training,** as they were the ones that showed statistical differences in the literature and in previous studies. It was therefore possible to establish a more substantive comparison of the results obtained.

The ***Kolmogorov-Smirnov and Shapiro-Wilk*** tests were used to determine the distribution of the variables in terms of symmetry and normality, and only the **Emotional Intelligence** variable and the **Self-Awareness** capacity were found to have a normal distribution. We therefore applied parametric analysis to the Emotional Intelligence and **Self-Awareness** variables, using the **Student's *t-test*** when crossing them with the dichotomous variables, and applied analysis of variance using the ***One Way* ANOVA test** with the Postgraduate Training variable. Non-parametric analysis was used for all the other skills and EI factors. In this case, when we wanted to analyze their relationship with the dichotomous characterization variables, we used the **Mann-Whitney *U-test*,** and with the postgraduate training variable we used the **Kruskal-Wallis test**.

In order to find out which variables influence the factors, skills and EI, we applied the tests with a probability of 95%, resulting in a significance level of 5%. This level of significance will allow us to affirm, with 95% *certainty,* the existence of a causal relationship between the variables. The decision criteria for confirming the relationship were based on the study of probabilities, confirming the relationship if the significance level was lower than 0.05 and rejecting it if it was higher than this value. The following significance levels were therefore taken into account:

- $p > 0.05$ - not significant;
- $p < 0.05$ - significant (95% confidence level);
- $p < 0.01$ - highly significant (99% confidence level);
- $p < 0.001$ - highly significant;
- $p < 0.0001$ - highly significant.

Finally, we carried out a correlational study and hierarchical multiple regression. According to Murteira (cited by Pestana and Gageiro, 2003, p.189), "Correlation indicates that phenomena are not indissolubly linked, but rather that the intensity of one is tended to be accompanied (on average, more frequently) by the intensity of the other, in the same direction or in the opposite direction." With the correlational analysis, we want to find out whether or not there is a correlation between the skills and the overall EI, as well as between all the factors that emerge from the sample of nurses and the EI skills and the overall EI. We also wanted to find the *strength* and *direction of* this relationship, as well as which ability has the highest correlation with global EI. To study the correlations, according to Pestana and Gageiro (2003), we assumed that a Pearson's r of less than 0.20 indicates a very low association; between 0.20 and 0.39 low; between 0.40 and 0.69 moderate; between 0.70 and 0.89 high and, finally, between 0.90 and 1.00 (one) a very high association. To calculate the correlations, the fully answered cases/questionnaires were used, using the bivariate correlation: *Exclude cases Listwise.*

Once we knew the relationship between the different variables, we tried to find out which variables were predictive of Emotional Intelligence, i.e. what contribution each variable made to predicting or explaining EI in this sample. In order to fulfill this objective, we carried out a hierarchical multiple regression, selecting the Stepwise method, as we considered it to be an option that guaranteed a better selection of the variables with the greatest predictive power (Pestana and Gageiro, 2003). For this procedure, only continuous variables should be used and, exceptionally, the dichotomous variable - gender - is also seen in some studies. There are no continuous variables in the characterization variables we used in our study. We therefore regressed only the EI abilities and the Gender variable on Emotional Intelligence, which is considered in this procedure to be the dependent variable. Linear regression was also carried out in order to establish the best possible prediction of the correlations between the variables under analysis and to investigate the percentage of variance that each of them presented.

Finally, with these operations, we have set ourselves the following objectives: to know if these scales measure what they intend to measure; to know if there are correlations between the constructs under study; to be able to make predictions (without obviously serving to infer causal relationships) and to know the distribution of correlation values in order of importance, according to the results of the sample studied.

Chapter 4

4 - MAIN RESULTS

This chapter will present the results obtained from the data collection. The results will be presented in the following order: characterization of the sample, factorial analysis of the subscales, descriptive analysis of the values of the variables (with the respective tests applied), correlational analysis and, finally, the presentation of the results of the study of the predictive variables of emotional intelligence.

In order to better interpret and analyze the data, we have used tables and charts, which will provide important support for the analysis of the statistical data obtained. Perhaps because it was optional to fill in the *other* item, there were very few responses. We therefore chose not to include them in the statistical analysis. The aim of the analysis of the open-ended questions was essentially to organize and synthesize the survey data so that we could identify other characteristics of EI skills that were not included in the respective sub-scales and were valued by each of the respondents. Therefore, as the responses given by the participants were not numerous, we did not carry out a qualitative analysis. However, these data were subjected to a floating reading, in an attempt to "make inferences, with an explicit logic, about the messages whose characteristics have been inventoried and systematized" (p.104), according to Vala (1989). This allowed us to get an overall impression of the responses obtained, with the questions relating to the Management of Emotions standing out, as they were the ones with the most responses overall. It was also found that there were free responses in all the sub-scales, with the exception of the Management of Relationships in Groups sub-scale. Some of the questions recorded by the sample are similar (from an interpretative point of view) to others that already make up the original questionnaire.

We will now break down (textually) the answers recorded by the participants in the study, grouping them according to the question they are on and the Lickert scale value assigned.

In the Self-Awareness sub-scale
Question I1 - Faced with a negative situation/relationship in my life, I feel that I get caught up in unpleasant feelings:
- "Later I think about what went wrong and what I could have done to improve my performance" - 7 (Q.45).

In the Emissions Management sub-scale
Question II1 - Imagine a situation in your life (personal or professional) in which you were overcome by a wave of fury or anger. Trying to calm down, you usually take action:
- "As soon as I had the chance, I faced the situation (person) and resolved it as best I could" - 4 (Q.45);
- "Talking to someone" - 5 (Q.136).

Question II2 - When, on a daily basis, I am invaded by negative emotions and feelings (fury, anger), I am usually..:

- "I do aqua aerobics" - 7 (Q.29);
- "I need to talk to someone, to 'defog' and accept what has happened" - 5 (Q.136).

Question II4 - When I feel depressed, I notice that:
- "I kill myself working even harder" - no answer (Q.98);
- "I eat out a lot" - 6 (Q.19);
- "I do anything that gives me pleasure" - 7 (Q.34);
- "I try to overlap these thoughts with leisure activities" - 6 (Q.62);
- "Talking to friends" - 7 (Q.63);
- "I do other activities that make me change these very negative behaviors" - 4 (Q.136);
- "I try to distract myself with positive situations in my life and overcome the depressive feeling" - 6 (Q.166);
- "I try to go out to distract myself" - 7 (Q.204).

In the Aiito-Motivaeao sub-scale

Question III2 - Imagine a professional activity (wound care, bladder catheterization, teaching the patient/family, etc.). During the activity, I usually feel that:
- "I feel satisfied and I improve my techniques" - 5 (Q.136).

Question III3 - When I experience personal rejection (intimately, socially, professionally), I feel that:
- "I try to come to a conclusion as to why this happened and I try to find out where the mistake is" - 6 (Q.166).

In the Empathy sub-scale

Question IV1 - In my relationships (personal, family, social) with others throughout my life, I get the feeling that I am capable of
of:
- "Tuning in to how they feel, even if they don't speak - no answer" (Q.63).

It should be noted that the responses to the optional items were spread over 10 questionnaires. This means that only 4.67% of respondents chose to answer these questions. This leads us to believe that the sample prefers to answer a scale of closed questions rather than open questions.

Despite being asked to fill in all the answers, of the 214 completed surveys, 17 were incomplete. However, we chose to include them in the analysis because the number of non-responses was not significant. In the case of the factorial analysis of the principal components, they took the value of the average of the responses to the item in question.

For methodological reasons, we will begin by characterizing the sample. The data found in the characterization of the sample may prove important for understanding the results obtained.

4.1- CHARACTERIZATION OF THE PROFESSIONALS

STUDIES

Bearing in mind that the target population for this study is 314 nurses (with a contractual relationship to an EPE Hospital), it can be seen that not all nurses were covered. We note that in the Operating Room Service, more than half of the nurses did not answer the questionnaire, giving a response rate of 24.5%. As this is one of the largest departments in the hospital, this considerably reduced the size of our sample.

Age and Gender

Table 1 shows a predominantly female group - 158 nurses (73.8% of the sample), with the most represented ages being between 21 and 30 years old, with 152 nurses (71% of the sample). The average age of the sample was 29.49 (SD=7.22).

Table 1 - Absolute and percentage cross-distribution of sample values according to age and gender

Age Gender	21-25 Years	26-30 Years	31-35 Years	36-40 Years	41-45 Years	46-50 Years	>51 Years	Total
Female	53 24,8%	54 25,2%	21 9,8%	11 5,1%	11 5,1%	5 2,3%	3 1,4%	158 73,8%
Male	20 9,3%	25 11,7%	4 1,9%	3 1,4%	2 0,9%	0 0%	2 0,9%	56 26,2%
T<tal	73 34,1%	79 36,9%	25 11,7%	14 6,5%	13 6,1%	5 2,3%	5 2,3%	214 100%

Academic qualifications and Immigrant

As far as academic qualifications are concerned, we found that Portuguese nurses have higher qualifications than foreign nurses. Of the total sample, 154 nurses are Portuguese (72%) and, of these, 109 nurses (50.9%) have a degree. Of the 60 immigrant nurses, who represent 28% of the total sample, only six (2.8%) have a degree.

All the immigrants mentioned are of Spanish nationality, with the exception of two participants. One is Cuban and the other has dual Spanish and Brazilian nationality.

Table 2 - Absolute and percentage cross-distribution of the sample in relation to the variables: Academic qualifications and Immigrant

Immigrant Academic qualifications	No		Yes		Total	
	N	%	N	%	N	%
Bachelor's degree	45	21,1	54	25,2	99	46,3
Degree	109	50,9	6	2,8	115	53,7
Total	154	72,0	60	28,0	214	100

Number of people in charge

71% of the nurses in the sample have no dependents (children or other dependents), probably because they are a very young group. There are 33 nurses with one dependent (15.4%) and the remaining 13.5% have between two and four dependents.

Table 3 - Absolute and percentage distribution of the sample in relation to the number of dependents

Number of people in charge	Total	
	N	%
0	152	71,0
1	33	15,4
2	18	8,4
3	5	2,3
4	6	2,8
Total	214	100

Graduate

From the analysis in Table 4, we can conclude that the vast majority of our sample of nurses do not have a postgraduate degree, representing 189 nurses (88.3%) of our total sample. It should be noted that 7% of our sample has a specialty.

Table 4 - Absolute and percentage distribution of the sample in relation to postgraduate training

Postgraduate training	Total	
	N	%
None	189	88,3
Specialty	15	7,0
Postgraduate studies	6	2,8
Master's student	2	0,9
Specialty + Master's student	1	0,5
Specialty + Postgraduate degree	1	0,5
Total	214	100

The postgraduate courses mentioned by the respondents were:

- Specialized Course in Rehabilitation Nursing;
- Specialization Course in Medical-Surgical Nursing;
- Specialization Course in Health Services Administration;
- Specialization Course in Child and Pediatric Health Nursing (two cases);
- Maternal Health and Obstetrics Nursing Specialization Course (10 cases);
- Postgraduate Course in Clinical Supervision (five cases);
- Postgraduate course in Health Pedagogy;
- Postgraduate course in Sports Nursing;
- Master's Degree in Education, Gender and Citizenship (to be attended);
- Master's Degree in Clinical Supervision (to be attended);

- *Unspecified* Master's course (to be attended).

Gender and Other Specific Training

The percentage of nurses who said they had undergone other relevant training was significantly low (8.4%), corresponding to
18 nurses. There were no major differences between the sexes (eight males and 10 females), as can be seen in the table below.

Table 5 - Absolute and percentage cross-distribution of the sample in relation to the variables: Gender and Other specific training

Gender Other specific training	Male		Female		Total	
	N	%	N	%	N	%
No	48	22,4	148	69,2	196	91,6
Yes	8	3,7	10	4,7	18	8,4
Total	56	26,1	158	73,9	214	100

Of the participants who answered *yes*, the following additional training took place:

- Advanced Life Support Course (three cases);
- Technical and Professional Course in Biotechnology;
- "Experto en Idosos" (Specialist - in Spanish);
- Postgraduate course in Health Marketing (frequency - incomplete);
- Master in Operating Room (Spanish, no translation);
- Pre-hospital, Resuscitation and Trauma Training Course;
- Course in Global Postural Re-education, Phenofibrolysis with hooks and Osteopathy;
- Degree in Educational Sciences (attendance - incomplete);
- Degree in Anthropology (attendance - incomplete);
- Human Resources Management Course and Leadership and Motivation Course;
- Palliative Care Training Course;
- Initial Pedagogical Training Course for Trainers (five cases).

Weekly working hours and professional category

With regard to professional category, the results are as follows: 154 nurses (71.9%) are level I nurses, 44 (20.6%) are graduates, 11 (5.1%) are specialists and four (1.8%) are managers.

From the table below, we can see that the vast majority of nurses work between 35 and 42 hours a week, with level I nurses working the most hours over 42.

Table 6 - Absolute cross-distribution of the variables: Weekly working hours and Professional category

Working hours Professional category	35-42	43-50	51-58	>59	Total

Nurse	120	17	11	6	154
Graduate	29	8	2	5	44
Specialist	9	1	1	0	11
Chief	4	1	0	0	5
Total	162	27	14	11	214

Contractual link

With regard to the type of contract each nurse has with the hospital, the results are as follows: 147 nurses (68.7%) have an open-ended contract, 39 nurses (18.2%) are on fixed-term contracts and 28 (13.1%) of the nurses in the sample are civil servants.

Table 7 - Absolute and percentage distribution of the sample in relation to the contractual relationship with the institution

Contractual link	Total	
	N	%
Fixed-term contract	39	18,2
Open-ended contract	147	68,7
Civil servant	28	13,1
Total	214	100

Time Served and Professional Achievement

With regard to professional fulfillment, we were curious to know if this varied with length of service/professional experience. We found that the vast majority of our sample felt fulfilled as nurses (192 nurses - 90.6%). This suggests that this fulfillment increases with length of service, as 17 (8%) of the 20 nurses (9.4%) who reported not feeling fulfilled as a nurse have been working for less than five years. However, it is worth noting that more than half of the nurses (64.6%) have been working for less than six years. Two nurses did not answer these two questions.

Table 8 - Absolute and percentage cross-distribution of the variables: length of service and professional achievement

Time of serv. Performed PrOf	0-5	6-10	11-15	16-20	21-25	26-30	>31	Total
No	17	0	0	3	0	0	0	20
	8%	0%	0%	1,4%	0%	0%	0%	9,4%
Yes	120	36	13	13	3	3	4	192
	56,6%	17%	6,1%	6,1%	1,4%	1,4%	1,9%	90,6%
Total	137	36	13	16	3	3	4	212
	64,6%	17%	6,1%	7,5%	1,4%	1,4%	1,9%	100%

Type of service

To get a more detailed idea of the distribution of nurses among the hospital's different services, we present the following tables.

Table 9 - Absolute and percentage distribution of the sample in relation to the Servigo variable

Served	Total	
	N	%
UCIP	16	7,5
Private Rooms	15	7,0
Surgery	25	11,7
Orthopedics	11	5,1
Obstetrics	13	6,1
Medicine	41	19,1
Oncology	6	2,8
Pediatrics	13	6,1
Operating Room	12	5,6
Pediatrics and Neonatology	1	0,5
Emergency and ICU	2	0,9
Neonatology	7	3,3
Birth Center	21	9,8
Urgency	22	10,3
JRC	1	0,5
UCI	8	3,7
Total	214	100

Regarding the distribution of the nurses under study among the hospital's services, 132 (62%) work in so-called *chronic services* and 81 nurses (38%) work in *acute services* (table 10). One nurse, who works in the Infection Control Committee (ICC), was excluded because he does not provide direct care to patients.

Table 10 - Absolute and percentage distribution of the sample, after transforming the Service variable into a dichotomous variable Type of service

Type of service	Total	
	N	%
Chronic	132	62,0
Acute	81	38,0
Total	213	100

Likes the workplace and considers it to have the right working conditions

With regard to the variable *Liking the workplace*, 212 (99.1%) nurses answered yes, 180 nurses (84.1%) said they had the right working conditions to carry out their duties and 33 nurses (15.4%) answered no.

Considers the interpersonal relationship with users important for the success of the care provided

With regard to this question, 154 nurses (72%) consider interpersonal relationships to be very important for the success of the care provided, 57 nurses (26.6%) consider them to be very important and there was only one response to each of the items: Indifferent (0.5%), Not very important (0.5%) and Not important (0.5%).

Table 11 - Absolute and percentage distribution of the sample regarding the level of importance of the interpersonal relationship with users for the success of the care provided

Interpersonal relationships with users for successful care	Total	
	N	%
Not important	1	0,5
Not very important	1	0,5
Indifferent	1	0,5
Very important	57	26,6
Very important	154	72,0
Total	214	100

Your ideas are listened to and put into practice

Regarding the question: *Do you feel that your ideas are listened to and put into practice*, 170 nurses (79.4%) say yes and 41 (19.2%) answer that their ideas are neither listened to nor put into practice.

Do you consider your emotional stability important in interpersonal relationships with others (users, multidisciplinary team, bosses, etc.)?

As for the importance of their emotional stability, we found that: 131 nurses (61.2%) consider it very important for interpersonal relationships, 81 nurses (37.8% of the sample) consider it quite important, and only one nurse (0.5%) considers it indifferent and another not very important (0.5%).

Table 12 - Absolute and percentage distribution of the sample regarding the level of importance of Emotional stability in interpersonal relationships

Emotional stability, important in interpersonal relationships	Total	
	N	%
Not important	0	0,0

Not very important	1	0,5
Indifferent	1	0,5
Very important	81	37,8
Very important	131	61,2
Total	214	100

You consider your relationships with people (family or social) to be important for your emotional stability.

In the table below, we can see that the relationship with other people is considered very important for their emotional stability by 123 nurses (57.5%), and quite important for 38.8% of nurses.

Table 13 - Absolute and percentage distribution of the sample regarding the level of importance of Relationships with people for emotional stability

Relationships with people, important for your emotional stability	Total	
	N	%
Not important	0	0,0
Not very important	2	0,9
Indifferent	6	2,8
Very important	83	38,8
Very important	123	57,5
Total	214	100

Throughout your experience as a nurse, do you consider that you have experienced the care process with levels of success?

With regard to this variable, the results are as follows: 122 nurses (57%) consider that they have experienced the care process at a fairly high level of success, 81 (37.9%) consider this success to be normal and nine nurses (4.7%) consider that they have experienced it at very high levels of success (table 14). Two nurses did not answer (one of them belongs to the CCI).

Today, you find it rewarding to be a nurse

It can be seen that the nurses who perceive the care process with the highest levels of success are precisely those who find their profession the most rewarding, as can be seen in the table below. Two nurses did not respond.

Table 14 - Absolute cross-distribution of the variables: Gratified to be a nurse and Experience of the care process with levels of success

Gratified to be a nurse Success in care	Nothing gratifying	Not very rewarding	Indifferente	Very gratifying	Very gratifying	Total
Very low	0	0	0	0	0	0
Bass	0	0	0	0	0	0
Normal	1	16	13	40	11	81
Quite high	0	10	8	72	32	122
Very high	0	1	0	4	4	9
Total	1	27	21	116	47	212

4.2 - SCALE CHARACTERISTICS

The set of items comprising each sub-scale was subjected to principal component factorial analysis - with Varimax scaling - to transform the expressions into groupable data or aggregation factors (tables 4 to 8). The purpose of using factorial analysis was to group the related items into main components or factors and to validate each sub-scale as independent constructs. Cronbach's alpha coefficient was used to measure the degree of internal consistency between the items and thus the level of reliability of each sub-scale.

The analysis was carried out on the basis of the principles previously defined (statistical treatment chapter). Thus, if the number of factors was close to the previous study in an exploratory way, we didn't force the rotation - in the case of the **Self-awareness**, **Emotion Management** and **Empathy** sub-scales. In the case of the **Managing Relationships in Groups** sub-scale, the number of factors in our sample was higher and so we forced it to the number of factors presented in the teacher validation. In the case of the **Automotivation** sub-scale, although the results of the exploratory analysis created the same number of factors as Augusta Branco's validation (four), it made more sense for us to force it to three, for reasons we will explain below. These procedures allowed us to construct 17 factors, identifying attitudes and behaviors related to EI, grouped into the sub-scales (which are intended for them), giving substance to each of the abilities.

All the factors found are integrated into the respective skills in tables 4, 5, 6, 7 and 8. **Four** factors were extracted from the **Self-awareness** sub-scale; **five factors** were extracted from the **Emotion Management sub-scale**; the **Self-motivation sub-scale** was forced into **three** factors; **three factors were** extracted from the **Empathy sub-scale**, and **two factors were** forced into the **Group Relationship Management** sub-scale.

4.3 - FACTORIAL SOLUTION OF THE SUB-SCALES

SELF-AWARENESS

The (exploratory) Factor Analysis carried out on **1ª capacity - Self-awareness** extracted four main factors, explaining 52.9% of the total variance, with a Cronbach's a value of 0.71 for the internal validity of the construct, selecting all 20 items from the sub-scale (table 2).

As can be seen in table 2, all the questions saturated above 0.30. But several questions saturated in more than one factor, so they were included where they saturated the most. These were *Mental retention of those feelings...; Positive, views life positively; Regardless of what they feel, they are sure of their limits; Clear awareness of what they feel, but do everything they can to keep them at bay; Identifies what they feel and can verbalize it.*

An exception was the question *Unlucky, unlucky in life*, which despite having a higher saturation in factor 5 (saturation=0.67), was kept in factor 1 (saturation=0.38) based on an analysis of the characteristics of its content. In this way, factor 5 was eliminated.

The dimensions (factors/components) that emerge from the grouping of items seem to measure the following aspects of Self-Awareness:

- The first factor, which we call ***Emotional Instability***, alone explains 17.9% of the total variance, with a Cronbach's a value of 0.83, which positively attests to the construct's internal validity.

This factor includes seven questions that reflect items related to emotional instability in the face of negative situations.

- The second factor explains 12.6% of the total variance of the sub-scale under analysis and has a Cronbach's a value of 0.81. The factor has good internal consistency, which is why it was named ***Changes at the rational and relational level***.

This factor combines three questions that reflect items related to changes in reasoning and relating to negative situations/relationships.

- The third factor, accounting for 12.4% of the total variance and a Cronbach's a value of 0.70, exposes the ***positive perception of oneself as a person***.

This factor combines five questions that reflect items related to positive self-recognition.

- The fourth factor, ***Perception of the occurrence of emotional phenomena, with a*** Cronbach's a value of 0.64, is representative of the factor's internal consistency, explaining 10% of the total variance.

This factor includes five questions that reflect items related to the perception of negative phenomena and their adaptive response.

We eliminated a fifth factor that contained two items, which for the reasons mentioned above were placed in two other factors.

Table 2 - Factorial solution of the Self-awareness sub-scale (1ª Capacity): Explained variance, Cronbach's alpha and item saturation value

ITEMS	Saturation
1st FACTOR (17.9%): F1 - Emotional instability - at 0.83	
- It absorbs itself, unable to escape, conditioning its behavior	0,77
- I fall into a negative state of mind, with *ruminations*	0,75
- If you're invaded by negative feelings, you can't control them	0,70

- He acts like a *ruminative* person, always mulling things over	0,68
- You're mentally stuck in these feelings...	0,60
- Unstable, with mood swings	0,56
- He's unlucky, unlucky in life	0,38

2nd FACTOR **(12.6%)**: **F2** - Rational and relational changes⁻ α **0,81**

- Altered attention span	0,83
- Decreases your level of reasoning	0,82
- Relational behavior changes	0,72

3rd FACTOR **(12.4%)**: **F3** - Positive perception of yourself as a person⁻ α **0,70**

- Flexible, adaptable to new ideas	0,73
- He's rational about his feelings	0,68
- He's observant, aware of what's going on around him	0,66
- Is autonomous, independent of fears and other opinions	0,65
- You're positive, you look at life positively	0,53

4th FACTOR **(10%)**: **F4** - Perception of the occurrence of emotional phenomena⁻ α **0,64**

- Right away, you become aware of your state of mind	0,77

- You have the exact notion of the type of feelings... you can define them	0,73
- No matter how he feels, he's sure of his limits	0,55
- Identifies what they feel and can verbalize it	0,46
- She's clearly aware of her feelings, but does everything she can to keep them at bay.	0,44
Total variance = **52.9%** overall Cronbach's = **0.71**	

EMOTION MANAGEMENT

The principal component analysis, which analyzes how the **2ª capacity**, *Management of Emotions* (table 3), was perceived by the sample subjects, extracts (in an exploratory way) five main subjects, extracted (in an exploratory way) five main factors which explained 57.3% of the total variance, with a Cronbach's a value of 0.69 showing reasonable internal validity of the construct.

Table 3 - Factorial solution of the Emotions Management sub-scale (2ª Capacity): Explained variance, Cronbach's alpha and item saturation value

ITEMS	Saturagao
1st FACTOR **(17.1%)**: **F5** - Negative adaptation (intrusion, explosion) - **at 0.80**	
- You have intrusive, persistent thoughts that haunt you	0,77
- Unconsciously, he uses more depressing thoughts	0,77
- He ends up isolating himself with no patience for anything	0,73
- Lives in a state of chronic worry	0,72
- He reacts, but without leaving the line of thought that worries him	0,64
- Uses objects, people or situations as targets for their anger	0,52
2nd FACTOR **(12.2%)**: **F6** - Control using reason - α **0,68**	

- Reason, try to understand and identify the origin	0,84
- Look at it from another angle, reassessing the cause	0,81
- He can see feelings, without judging, and start thinking positively	0,63
- Stay alert: identify the negative emotion, examine and re-evaluate it	0,50
3rd FACTOR (9.5%): F7 - Escape and loneliness - α 0,53	
- Calms down in an unprovoked environment	0,82
- Look for a distraction	0,62
- He's alone, looking for calm	0,62
4th FACTOR (9.4%): F8 - Anxious, reactive feelings - α 0,59	
- He's distressed, trying to catch his worries as soon as possible	0,72
- Perceiving dangers... and thinking about them is a way of dealing with them	0,72
- He worries, but diverts attention from his negative state of mind	0,68
5th FACTOR (9.1%): F9 - Control by physical activity - α 0,70	
- Do active physical exercise	0,88
- You feel relief if you do intense sport	0,83
Total variance = 57.3% α Overall Cronbach's = 0.69	

As you can see, all of the questions reach saturations of either

above 0.50, and none of the 18 items relating to this ability were rejected. It should be noted that, in this sub-scale, there was only one question - *Worry, but diverting attention from these emotions* - which saturated in two factors, so it was included where it saturated the most.

These factors seem to measure the following aspects of emotion management:

- The first factor, which explains 17.1% of the variance and whose internal validity of the construct is 0.80, was called ***Negative Adaptation (intrusion, explosion)***.

This factor combines six questions that group together attitudes and behaviors of negative adaptation, with negative thoughts and reactions.

- The second factor, which accounts for 12.2% of the variance in the total sub-scale, has an internal validity value of (a 0.68). These values presuppose a good consistency of this factor, which is called *Control using the ratio*.

The factor combines four questions that reflect items related to the rationalization of emotions and negative feelings.

- The third factor, called *Escape and loneliness*, already has a lower percentage of variance (9.5%) and the lowest value for the construct's internal validity (0.53), but it still has an acceptable internal consistency.

This factor combines three questions that reflect items related to adaptation mechanisms, through isolation and distraction from other subjects.

- The fourth factor, explaining 9.4% of the total variance and with a value of a 0.59, was called *Anxious, reactive feelings*.

This factor associates three questions that group together attitudes and reaction behaviors and ways of dealing with anxiety.

- Finally, the fifth factor, called *Control by physical activity*, explains 9.1% of the total variance and has an internal consistency value of 0.70.

The factor combines two questions that reflect the control of your emotions through physical activity.

AUTOMOTIVATION

In the analysis of the results obtained in the exploratory factorial solution carried out on the **3ª capacity**, *Self-motivation*, the original 21 items were kept and four factors emerged. It seemed to us that the factors - one and three - tended to be grouped together, and that all the items saturated in the two factors (although more in one than the other), we tried a forced factorial analysis of three factors. In this way, and after rotation, these two factors grouped exactly into one, which, by the way, was the one where the items had the highest factorial weight. We therefore opted for this factorial solution, which seemed to us to be the most appropriate, having previously defined three main factors, despite the fact that Branco's validation (1999) presented four factors.

There were two questions that saturated in more than one factor, so they were included where they saturated the most. These were: *The more creative the work, the more you absorb it* and You *experience feelings of pleasure (personal enjoyment)*.

Thus, the three main factors found explain 46.2% of the total variance (table 4), with a Cronbach's a value of 0.75 confirming the construct's internal validity. All the items show saturation above 0.40.

Table 4 - Factorial solution of the Automotivation sub-scale (3ª Capacity): Variance explained, Cronbach's alpha and item saturation value

ITEMS	Saturagao

50

1st FACTOR (22.5%): F10 - Illiterate, insecure and dependent - α **0,86**	
- You're invaded by self-pity	0,71
- You're overwhelmed by anxiety and frustration	0,67
- He's in a bad mood, invaded only by negative memories	0,67
- Feeling pessimistic (whatever you do will go wrong)	0,66
- He is invaded by contempt and resentment	0,65
- Feeling defeatist (unlucky in life)	0,65
- You're plagued by thoughts: won't they like it?	0,64
- Thinks it's a personal flaw, "I'm like that"	0,64
- Think about it and ruminate on the humiliation	0,62
- You're making and ruminating on other thoughts	0,59
- You're doing what you have to, with a worried state of mind	0,56
2nd FACTOR (15.2%): F11 - Literates use emotional energy - α **0,76**	
- Is capable of having the energy and ability to tackle problems	0,78
- He doesn't mind waiting, even in challenging situations	0,70
- Control your impulses - act after thinking	0,67
- Is flexible enough to change objectives if they prove impossible	0,66
- He can get out of any trouble	0,57
- The more creative the work, the more it absorbs you	0,49

- You think of a fact and find a contemporizing attitude	0,48
3rd FACTOR **(8.5%)**: **F12** - "Flow status" in activity (assets) - α **0,58**	
- Lose track of time and space	0,81
- He is absolutely absorbed, indifferent to his surroundings	0,80
- Experiencing sensations of pleasure (personal enjoyment)	0,43
Total variance = **46.2%** α Overall Cronbach's = **0.75**	

The groupings of the items in the Self-motivation sub-scale seem to measure the following domains:

- The items saturated in the first factor, called *Illiterates, with insecurity and dependence*, alone explain 22.5% of the variance and have an internal construct validity value (at 0.86) representative of the factor's internal coherence.

This factor combines eleven questions that bring together attitudes and personal perceptions of low self-motivation, insecurity and passivity.

- The second factor, which explains 15.2% of the total variance and has a Cronbach's a value of 0.76 (well representative of the factor's internal consistency), is called *Literates, they use emotional energy.*

The factor combines seven questions that reflect items related to the existence of the Self-Motivation skill.

- The third factor, with the lowest variance (8.5%) and a value of 0.58, is called *"State of flow" in activity (assets)*. This is one of the factors with the lowest value in terms of the construct's internal validity.

Here, three questions are linked which reflect items related to attitudes of optimism and activity.

EMPATHY

As can be seen in table 5, the exploratory factorial analysis extracted 11 items distributed across three factors from the 12 items that made up the **4ª capacity** - *Empathy*. These explained 60.2% of the total variance and a Cronbach's a value of 0.83, which suggests the construct's internal validity.

All questions saturated above 0.30.

As can be seen in table 5, in this sub-scale there were two questions that saturated more than one factor, so they were included where they saturated more. These were *The direction of the gaze* and *Reading non-verbal channels*.

An exception was made for the question "*Tuning in to the feelings of others if they use clarifying words*". Although this question has a factor loading of 0.46 in factor 1, it was decided to include it in factor 2 (where it saturates with 0.34). This choice was based on an analysis of the characteristics of its content.

Table 5 - Factorial solution of the Empathy sub-scale (4ª Capacity): Variance explained, Cronbach's alpha and item saturation value

ITEMS	Saturagao
1st FACTOR **(27%)**: **F13** - Values expression (verbal and non-verbal) - α **0,83**	
- Enhance your tone of voice	0,84
- Value gestures (hands, body)	0,78
- Enhances the direction of the gaze	0,76
- Value the consonance between words and the person's body attitude	0,70
- Appreciates the verbal expression of others	0,67
2nd FACTOR **(16.8%)**: **F14** - Relational harmony - α **0,68**	
- Is attuned to the feelings of others, regardless of verbal expression	0,76
- Registers / perceives feelings	0,71
- Read the non-verbal channels	0,71
- You tune in to other people's feelings if they use enlightening words	0,34
3rd FACTOR **(16.5%)**: **F15** - Serene attitude in conflict situations - α **0,75**	
- Use calm to listen	0,81
- Is receptive to instability with a calm attitude	0,79
Total variance = **60.2%** α Overall Cronbach's = **0.83**	

Also, after rotation, the item - *Receptivity to instability with an unstable attitude* - saturated negatively (-0.68) in the third factor. Its content was recoded and analyzed, and it was noted that its interpretative value was similar to another item (*Receptivity to instability with a serene attitude* - from the same factor). For this reason, and because the sample seemed to consider it *confusing and* not measuring their attitudes in the same circumstances, the item was eliminated. It should be noted that, by choosing this measure, the factor's a-value increased significantly from 0.69 to 0.75. The a-value of the sub-scale increased from 0.82 to 0.83.

Thus, the dimensions found seem to measure the following aspects of Empathy:

- The items saturated in the 1st factor alone explain 27% of the total variance of the sub-scale and the value of 0.83 refers to the internal validity of the construct.

This factor combines five questions that denote an attitude oriented towards emotional expression, which is why it has been called *Values expression (verbal and non-verbal)*.

- The second factor explains 16.8% of the variance and is representative (at 0.68) of the construct's internal validity.

This factor, called *Relational Attunement,* combines four questions that reflect items related to relational feelings: personal, family and social.

- The third factor explains 16.5% of the total variance and the value in relation to the internal validity of the construct is 0.75.

The factor combines two questions that reflect attitudes towards conflict situations, which is why it was called *Serene Attitude in Conflict Silence*.

GROUP RELATIONSHIP MANAGEMENT

In order to confirm the construct validity of this sub-scale, we carried out a factorial analysis of the 14 items of the **5ª capacity** - *Managing Relationships in Groups* (table 6) - with the prior definition of two factors. These explained 46.5% of the total variance, with a Cronbach's a value of 0.85.

Table 6 - Factorial solution of the Group Relationship Management sub-scale (5ª Capacity): Variance explained, Cronbach's alpha and item saturation value

ITEMS	Saturation
1st FACTOR **(26.8%)**: F16 - Emotional perception and synchronism - α **0,84**	
- Get in sync with your state of mind	0,79
- Makes the same gestures or gestures in agreement with the other person	0,73
- She picks up on other people's feelings and seems to start absorbing them	0,71
- Has an innate sensitivity to recognizing feelings	0,70
- You feel physically synchronized with those around you	0,61

- You understand how people are feeling	0,53
- Gives verbal expression to collective feelings	0,52
- Recognizes the feelings of others and acts to influence them	0,52
- You adjust to the feelings you read, without being liked	0,44
- Prefers to be face-to-face	0,39
2nd FACTOR (19.7%): F17 - Personal and relational stability - α 0,70	
• You have control over your own feelings	0,73
• Have stable personal relationships and maintain them over time	0,71
• In your relationships, you say what you think, regardless of other opinions...	0,63
• Control the expression of your own emotions	0,62
Total variance = **46.5%** α Overall Cronbach's = **0.85**	

The choice to increase the number of factors is also due to the fact that, in the first exploratory rotation with four factors, it was found that two of them included almost all of the items in the sub-scale and, furthermore, it is in line with the factorial solution found in the validation of the original scale for teachers carried out by Branco in 1999. Thus, in this sub-scale, the forgone rotation selects all the items from the theoretical proposal, and the sample did not consider any items that could cause confusion, i.e. no items were eliminated.

As can be seen (table 6), all the questions saturated above 0.30. It should be noted that in this sub-scale, there were several questions that saturated in more than one factor, so they were included where they saturated the most. These were: *Innate sensitivity to recognize feelings; Perceives how people are feeling; Gives verbal expression to collective feelings; Recognizes the feelings of others and acts to influence them and Adjusts to the feelings you read, other than to be liked.*

The components found seem to measure the following aspects of Group Relationship Management:

- The first factor explains 26.8% of the variance and the Cronbach's a value (0.84) positively attests to the validity of this factor. It associates 10 questions that reflect items related to the way the sample perceives their group relationships, which is why it is called Emotional perception and synchronism.

- The second factor, which explains 19.7% of the variance and has a Cronbach's a value of 0.70 (representative of the factor's internal consistency), combines four items that express the dominance that exists, or that they think exists, in their relationships, calling it *Personal and relational stability*.

Of the 85 items in the five sub-scales, only one item was eliminated. This procedure made it possible to construct 17 factors, which are grouped into the five EI capacities. Each factor integrates the respective ability it relates to: - the Self-awareness sub-scale has four factors, - the Emotion Management sub-scale has five, - the Self-motivation sub-scale has three factors, - the Empathy sub-scale has three and - the Group Relationship Management sub-scale has two factors.

Overall (at the level of the five sub-scales), the scale used showed good psychometric characteristics and alpha values considered acceptable, suggesting its reliability for use in this study.

4.4 - THE VALUES OF THE VARIABLES UNDER STUDY

In this section of the study, the values of the sample's answers will be analyzed in relation to: the factors extracted by the previous analysis, each of the EI abilities and the level of overall emotional intelligence. We will also present the distribution of the sample's responses, corresponding the values of the actual sums to the Likert scale used (table 7).

We will also check whether there are statistically significant differences with regard to some of the characterization variables we have selected.

Table 7 - Distribution of factors, abilities and Emotional Intelligence: Minimum-Maximum of responses (Min-Max), mean (X), standard deviation (SD) and weighted mean (MP)

	Capacities/Factors	Min/Max	X	(DP)	MP
	Self-awareness	**56-112**	**81,06**	**(10,18)**	**4,05**
F1	Emotional instability	9-38	19,96	(6,48)	2,85
F2	Rational and relational changes	3-21	10,31	(3,58)	3,44
F3	Positive perception of oneself as a person	15-35	25,55	(4,00)	5,11
F4	Perception of the occurrence of emotional phenomena	15-34	25,24	(4,13)	5,05
	Fire Management	**27-87**	**63,85**	**(9,56)**	**3,55**
F5	Negative adaptation (intrusion, explosion)	6-35	16,63	(5,72)	2,77

F6	Control using reason	4-26	16,03	(3,53)	4,01
F7	Escape and loneliness	3-21	12,91	(2,95)	4,30
F8	Anxious, reactive feelings	4-20	11,99	(2,80)	4,00
F9	Control by physical activity	2-14	6,27	(2,94)	3,14
	Automotive	**41-106**	**72,08**	**(10,03)**	**3,43**
F1	Illiterate, insecure and dependent	12-57	28,40	(8,33)	2,58
F1	Literates use emotional energy	19-48	33,45	(5,06)	4,78
F1	"Flow status" in activity (assets)	3-18	10,23	(3,11)	3,41
	Empathy	**37-75**	**53,53**	**(7,49)**	**4,87**
F1	Values expression (verbal and non-verbal)	12-35	24,8C	(4,38)	4,96
F1	Relational harmony	12-28	19,39	(3,14)	4,85
F1	A calm attitude in conflict situations	4-14	9,34	(2,03)	4,67
	Group Relationship Management	45-89	61,91	(8,58)	4,42
F1	Emotional perception and synchronism	27-61	42,60	(6,72)	4,26
F1	Personal and relationship stability	11-28	19,31	(3,23)	4,83
	Emotional Intelligence	**253-419**	**332,4**	**(32,59)**	**3,96**

Self-awareness

The first capacity has an average of 81.06 and a sample distribution between 71.42 and 91.24 (X ± 1DP), which corresponds (using the weighted average) to the Likert time scale - As a *rule*. The percentile table also shows that the sample has distributions between the 5th and 95th percentiles (between the values 66 and 99.10 - respectively), although 50% of the answers are between the 25th and 75th percentiles.

For the Self-awareness ability, the data does not suggest statistically significant differences in relation to any of the selected characterization variables. As for the factors that make up this ability, the data suggests that only factors 3 and 4 show statistical differences with the age variable.

Factor 1 has an average of 19.96 and sample distribution values of between 13.48 and 26.44 (X ± 1DP), which corresponds (on the Likert time scale) to **Rarely**, with a strong tendency towards *Infrequently*.

Factor 2 (with an average of 10.31) has a distribution between the values of 6.73 and 13.89 (X ± 1DP), which correspond to the attribution of **Infrequent**.

Factor 3 has an average of 25.55 and a sample distribution between 21.55 and 29.55 (X ± 1DP), placed at **Frequent**.

There are highly significant differences between this factor and the **age of** the nurses (Z = - 3.459; p = 0.001), suggesting that younger nurses (<40 years) have a lower positive perception of themselves as a person than older ones (Mean *Rank* = 101.84 and 145.13, respectively).

Factor 4, with an average of 25.24, lies between the values 21.11 and 29.37 (X ± 1DP). It assumes correspondence (weighted average) in **Frequent**.

The factor is significantly influenced by **age** (Z = -2.356; p = 0.018), as the data suggests that nurses aged 40 or over (Mean *Rank* = 131.88) have a higher perception of the occurrence of emotional phenomena than their younger colleagues (Mean *Rank* = 102.64).

Managing Emotions

The second capacity shows an average of 63.85 and a sample distribution between 54.29 and 73.41 (X ± 1 SD). By corresponding the scores to the Likert time scale, we can say that the weighted average is **Infrequent**, with a tendency towards As a *rule*. In the percentile table, the sample varies between the values 48.90 and 80.10 (of the 5th and 95th percentiles, respectively). However, 50% of the answers are between the 25th and 75th percentiles.

In this capacity, no statistically significant differences were found for any of the characterization variables used.

Factor 5 (mean 16.63) is distributed between values 10.91 and 22.35 (X ± 1 SD), situated in **Rarely,** with a strong tendency towards *Infrequently*.

Factor 6 has an average of 16.03 and a distribution of average sample values between 12.50 and 19.56 (X ± 1DP). The values correspond to the time frequency assignment of **By norm**.

There are highly significant differences between this factor and **age** (Z = - 2.636; *p = 0.008),* indicating that older nurses (Mean *Rank* = 135.50) have greater control *using the ratio* than younger ones (Mean *Rank* = 102.69).

Factor 7, with a mean value of 12.91, shows a distribution of sample mean values between 9.96 and 15.86 (X ± 1DP), which are within the **norm**.

Factor 8 (mean 11.99) has a sample distribution between the values 9.19 and 14.79 (X ± 1SD), which correspond to the attribution **By norm**.

Factor 9 has an average of 6.27, with average distribution curve values between 3.33 and 9.21 (X ± 1DP), which are in the **infrequent** range.

Gender has a significant influence on this factor (Z = -2.158; *p* = 0.031), as male nurses have greater (Mean *Rank* = 120.01) *control over physical activity* compared to female nurses (Mean *Rank* = 99.64).

Automotive

The third skill has an overall average of 72.08 and a sample distribution between 62.05 and 82.11 (X ± 1DP). Using the weighted average, we can match these values to the Likert scale distribution - *Infrequent*. The percentile table confirms the distribution between the values of 56 and 91.20 (corresponding to the 5th and 95th percentiles), with 50% of the answers falling between the 25th and 75th percentiles.

The data suggest that the selected characterization variables do not influence this variable.

Factor 10 (mean of 28.40) shows a distribution of the sample's mean values between 20.07 and 36.73 (X ± 1 SD), placing it at *Rarely* - with a tendency towards *Infrequent*.

The data suggests that nurses under the age of 40 (Mean *Rank* = 109.47) perceive themselves to be more insecure and dependent than older nurses (Mean *Rank* = 69.73). The *age* variable therefore has a highly significant influence on this factor of self-motivation ($Z = -3.152; p = 0.002$).

Factor 11 (mean 33.45) is distributed between values 28.39 and 38.51 (X ± 1SD), and is in the range of *Usually* - with a strong tendency towards *Often*.

The data suggests that there are statistically significant differences between this factor and *age* ($Z = -3.074; p = 0.002$). Younger nurses (Mean *Rank* = 99.05) perceive themselves as less able to use their emotional energy than older nurses (Mean *Rank* = 136.98).

Factor 12 has an average of 10.23 and a distribution of the sample values between 7.12 and 13.34 (X ± 1DP), which is in the *infrequent* range.

Empathy

The fourth capacity has an average of 53.53 and a distribution of sample values between 46.04 and 61.02 (X ± 1DP). These values are on the time frequency scale As a *rule* - with a strong tendency towards *Frequent*. The percentile table shows that the answers are distributed between the 5th and 95th percentiles (with values between 42 and 66.10), with 50% of the answers being between the 25th and 75th percentiles.

Age significantly influences the capacity for empathy ($Z = - 2.231; p = 0.026$). Nurses under the age of 40 perceive themselves as less empathetic (Mean *Rank* = 99.83) than older nurses (Mean *Rank* = 126.84).

Factor 13 has an average of 24.80 and a distribution of values between 20.42 and 29.18 (X ± 1DP), which are *Normal* - with a strong tendency towards *Frequent*.

Factor 14 (mean of 19.39) has a sample distribution between 16.25 and 22.53 (X ± 1SD), which fall within the range of As a *rule* - with a strong tendency towards *Frequent*.

The data suggests that there are statistically significant differences between *age* and this factor ($Z = -2.339; p = 0.019$), showing that younger nurses (Mean *Rank* = 100.16) feel less able to establish relational attunement than nurses aged 40 or over (Mean *Rank* = 128.52).

Factor 15 has an average value of 9.34. It has a sample mean distribution of between 7.31 and 11.37 (X ± SD), which is placed (on the Likert scale) in the As a *rule* - with a tendency towards *Frequent*.

The data suggests that there are statistically significant differences between the *type of service* and the factor ($Z = -2.025; p = 0.043$). Thus, nurses who work in services known as *chronic*

(Mean *Rank* = 111.99) use more calm and serenity when faced with conflict situations than nurses who work in services known as *acute* (Mean *Rank* = 94.74).

Group Relationship Management

The fifth EI ability has an overall average value of 61.91 and a sample distribution between 53.33 and 70.49 (X ± 1SD). By calculating the weighted average, we can match these values to the Likert time scale - *As a rule*. The percentile table shows a sample distribution of values between 49 and 78, obtained from the 5th percentile up to the 95th percentile. It also specifies that 50% of the results are between 56 and 67, i.e. between the 25th and 75th percentiles.

This ability is influenced by *age*, as the data shows that there are statistically significant differences (Z = - 2.904; *p* = 0.004). Thus, younger nurses perceive themselves as having greater difficulty in managing relationships (Mean *Rank* = 99.72) than older nurses (Mean *Rank* = 135.20).

With regard to *academic qualifications*, **we** also found highly significant statistical differences (Z = -2.748; *p* = 0.006). The data suggests that graduate nurses perceive themselves as more capable (Mean *Rank* = 115.11) in this capacity than nurses with a bachelor's degree (Mean *Rank* = 92.13).

We also found statistically significant differences between this ability and the *type of service* (Z = -2.046; p = 0.041). The data suggests that nurses working in *chronic* services also manage relationships better (Mean *Rank* = 110.62) than those working in *acute* services (Mean *Rank* = 93.06).

Factor 16 (mean of 42.60) shows a distribution of responses from the sample between 35.88 and 49.32 (X ± 1SD), which fall within the *By norm*.

In this factor, there were highly significant statistical differences in relation to *age* (Z = - 2.645; *p* = 0.008). Thus, the data suggests that nurses under the age of 40 (Mean *Rank=100*.65) have lower emotional perception and synchronism with others than older nurses (Mean *Rank=133*.09).

Academic qualifications also have a significant influence on this factor (Z = -2.567; p = 0.010). The data show that nurses with a university degree (Mean *Rank* = 114.88) are better at perceiving their emotions and synchrony than nurses with a bachelor's degree (Mean *Rank* = 93.36).

Factor 17 (mean value of 19.31) has mean distribution values for the sample between 16.08 and 22.54 (X ± 1DP), which fall within the range of As a *rule* - with a strong tendency towards *Frequent*.

There are statistically significant differences between this factor and *age* (Z = -2.711; p = 0.007). Thus, younger nurses (Mean *Rank* = 101.06) show less personal and relational stability than older nurses (Mean *Rank* = 134.34).

Academic qualifications also have a statistically significant influence on this factor (Z = - 2.182; p = 0.029). The data suggests that nurses with a bachelor's degree (Mean *Rank* = 114.02) perceive themselves as having greater personal stability and stability in the relationships they establish than those with a bachelor's degree (Mean *Rank*

= 95,77).

There were also statistically significant differences between the factor and the *type of service* (Z = -2.545; p = 0.011). Thus, the data seems to indicate that nurses who work predominantly in *acute* services (Mean *Rank* = 91.27) self-perceive personal and relational stability less often than nurses in *chronic* services (Mean *Rank* = 113.18).

Emotional Intelligence

The ***Emotional Intelligence*** variable (with an average global sum value of 332.44) shows a sample distribution between 299.85 and 365.03 (X ± 1SD). By calculating the weighted average, we can correspond these values to the Likert time scale assignment ***Infrequent*** - with a strong tendency towards *As a rule*. The percentile table shows a distribution of the sample starting at the 5th percentile, ranging from 275.9 to 388.10. With regard to the location, 50% of the answers are between the 25th and 75th percentiles, with values varying between 312 and 353.

In this variable, which is the sum of all the previous ones, we found that there are statistically significant differences between Emotional Intelligence and the ***type of service*** (t = 2.136; GL = 194; p = 0.034). The data suggests that nurses working in the type of service known as *chronic services* perceive themselves as having higher emotional intelligence skills (X = 336.22) than nurses working in *acute* services (X = 325.94).

With regard to the ***immigrant*** variable, it is important to note that, although 28.04% (60 nurses) are immigrants, there are no statistically significant differences between immigrant and Portuguese nurses with regard to the factors skills and Emotional Intelligence.

We also found no statistically significant differences in the ***postgraduate training*** variable.

Once these results are known, it will be interesting to know the correlation between the capabilities of the EI, as well as between these and the overall EI.

4.5 - CORRELATIONAL ANALYSIS

As mentioned above, the correlational analysis aims to find out whether or not there is a correlation between the abilities and the overall EI. We also want to find out the *strength* and direction of this relationship, as well as which ability has the highest correlation with overall Emotional Intelligence. To this end, Pearson's r coefficient will be used to obtain precise data on the relationship between the abilities and each other, as well as the relationship between the abilities and Emotional Intelligence.

In the table below, we can see that there is a statistically significant correlation between all the variables, confirming the positive relationship between them, i.e. the variation between the variables is in the same direction, with significant correlations for an overall significance level of p <0.01.

Table 8 shows that Empathy correlates moderately (r 0.653) with Managing Relationships in Groups, as does Managing Emotions with Self-awareness (r 0.492) and Self-motivation (r 0.571).

The same happens (r 0.511) between self-awareness and self-motivation. It should be noted that Empathy and Managing Relationships in Groups are the skills with the highest inter-skill correlation of all (r 0.653). There were no very low associations (< 0.20), which suggests that there is at least a low relationship between all the skills.

Table 8 - Distribution of correlations between abilities and Emotional Intelligence: Pearson's correlation (r) and significance level (p)

Variables		Self-awareness	Managing Emotions	Automotive	Empathy	Group Relationship Management
Fire Management	**r** **P**	**0,492** 0,000				
Automotive	r p	**0,511** 0,000	**0,571** 0,000			
Empathy	r p	0,211 0,003	0,261 0,000	0,297 0,000		
Group Relationship Management	r p	0,215 0,002	0,261 0,000	0,283 0,000	**0,653** 0,000	
Emotional Intelligence	r p	**0,719** 0,000	**0,751** 0,000	**0,777** 0,000	**0,636** 0,000	**0,645** 0,000

With regard to overall *Emotional Intelligence*, it shows a statistically significant high (> 0.70) and positive correlation with the subscales of the abilities: *Self-awareness* (r 0.719), *Management of Emotions* (r 0.751) and *Self-motivation* (r 0.777) and moderate with the skills of *Empathy (r 0*.636) and *Management of Relationships in groups (r 0*.645).

These data indicate that the sub-scales are related to Emotional Intelligence and that they measure the dimensions/capabilities of EI. The EI of the sample of nurses, according to their perception, shows the strongest positive correlations with: **1st -** *Self-motivation*, **2nd -** *Managing emotions,* **3rd -** *Self-awareness*, **4th -** *Managing relationships in groups* and, finally, **5th -** *Empathy* (with a correlation value of 0.636) - suggesting that this ability has the least influence on nurses' Emotional Intelligence. The way in which the abilities correlate with the dependent variable is different from that proposed in the theoretical construct, as can be seen in the next table.

4.5.1 - The theoretical construct Versus the sample responses

The correlational analysis presented below aims to compare Goleman's (2000, 2003) theoretical construct with the configuration of Emotional Intelligence found in the sample of nurses studied. In other words, the emotional competence of the nurses studied is mirrored here.

The analysis of the correlational study - construct *Versus* sample response - offers two moments for reflection. The first moment (left side of chart 9) reveals the correlational and schematic construction according to Goleman's (2000, 2003) theoretical construct, in which the sample, corroborating the author, shows the perception of behaviors and attitudes that correlate, more or less significantly, with each of the abilities. In other words, the five capacities of the theoretical model correlate positively and significantly with the dependent variable (Emotional Intelligence), and each of these capacities aggregates specific sets of behaviors and attitudes (items), which are more or less significantly correlated with these same capacities.

Table 9 - Comparative distribution of the magnitude of the correlations (Pearson's r) between the variables: factors, abilities and Emotional Intelligence, according to the theoretical construct and the sample responses ($p<0.01$)

THEORETICAL CONSTRUCT					SAMPLE ANSWERS			
Factors	r	Capabilities	r		r	Skills	r	Factors
							0,769	F10
F1	0,692				0,777	Automotive	0,607	F12
F2	0,630	Self-awareness					0,591	F5
F3	0,316		0,719				0,486	F1
F4	0,527						0,647	F5
							0,548	F8
					0,751		0,537	F7
F5	0,647					Fire Management	0,525	F10
F6	0,398			E			0,452	F9
F7	0,537		0,751	M			0,692	F1
F8	0,548	Fire Management		O			0,630	F2
F9	0,452			T	0,719	Self-awareness	0,527	F4
				I			0,463	F5
				O			0,428	F10
F10	0,769			N			0,562	F13
F11	0,341	Automotive	0,777	A	0,688		0,538	F14
F12	0,607			L		F16 – Perception	0,532	F11
						and Synchronism	0,414	F17

						0,939	F16
						0,701	F17
F13	0,867					0,625	F11
		Empathy	0,636	0,645		0,537	F13
F14	0,810					0,531	F14
F15	0,566				Group Relationship Management	0,489	F3
						0,431	F15
						0,404	F6
						0,867	F13
F16	0,939					0,810	F14
			0,645			0,658	F16
F17	0,701					0,566	F15
				0,636	Empathy	0,544	F11
		Group Relationship Management				0,437	F3
						0,416	F4

The lowest correlations are found between the *Self-awareness skill* and the *F3* factor (r 0, 316); the *Emotions Management skill* and the *F6 factor* (r 0.398) and the *Self-motivation* skill and the *F11* factor (r 0.341). The only very high correlation is between the ability to *Manage Relationships in Groups* and factor *F16* (r 0.939). All the other *factor-capability* associations are at moderate and high levels.

In the first three skills that are positively and highly associated with *Emotional Intelligence,* emerging from the subjects' responses, factors *F5* and *F10 are repeated,* as they show significant correlations. The *F1* factor is repeated between the *Self-awareness* and *Self-motivation* abilities.

In the second part of table 9 (right-hand side of the table), and respecting the values and respective statistical significance of the correlational study, in which all the variables under study - factors, abilities and *Emotional Intelligence* - are called upon to reveal the magnitude of their interaction with each other, we now have access to a new configuration for constructing the EI profile. In other words, the latter is the profile revealed through the sample's responses, which constitutes the emotional competence of the nurses studied. Here we are no longer studying each ability in isolation, but looking at all the variables in interaction (factors, abilities and EI).

Considering this second unit of analysis, which concerns the validation of the instrument based on the sample's responses and the respective level of inter-variable correlation, we can consider, from an overall perspective, that all the factors, EI abilities and Emotional Intelligence show positive and significant correlations, but not as recommended in the theoretical construct. The weakest correlations are found at the positive correlation level - moderate (r>0.40) - and there are no *factor-capability* associations at the low or very low level.

In this second grouping, there are three factors (*F11*, *F13* and *F14*) that are repeatedly associated with the two skills and factor *F16*. Between the skills of *Relationship Management in Groups* and *Empathy*,

the factors *F3* and F15 are repeated.

A more in-depth analysis of the data emerging from this framework of correlations will be made in the chapter discussing the results, in order to avoid repeating information. We would just like to highlight the fact that the sample included factor *F16* (*Emotional Perception and Synchronism*) with the most significant positive association (r 0.688) between the factors and Emotional *Intelligence*, an association that was slightly higher (at a moderate level) than that found between the skills of *Empathy* and *Relationship Management in Groups* and *Emotional Intelligence.*

Once we know the relationship between the variables - factors, abilities and Emotional Intelligence - we will try to find out which variables are predictive of Emotional Intelligence, in other words, what contribution each variable makes to predicting or explaining Emotional Intelligence in this sample.

4.6 - EXPLANATORY VARIABLES OF INTELLIGENCE NURSES' EMOTIONS

In order to find out the contribution of each variable to predicting or explaining Emotional Intelligence in this sample, we carried out a stepwise regression analysis for *Emotional Intelligence* (dependent variable), with only the variables - EI abilities and *gender* - being considered for regression.

The hierarchical regression analysis selected four independent variables, excluding *Empathy* and *gender,* as they did not present significant levels.

Table 10 - Stepwise regression analysis of abilities and gender for the dependent variable (p<0.05): Prediction/explanation values (adjusted R2), Determinate coefficients (ß), F statistic, degrees of freedom (GL) and significance levels (p).

Predictive variables	Adjusted R2	F (GL) p	P (P)
Automotive	0,60	297,67 (1-195) 0,000	0,77 (0,000)
Manage Group Relationships	0,79	388,48 (2-194) 0,000	0,46 (0,000)
Self-awareness	0,91	658,78 (3-193) 0,000	0,39 (0,000)

Fire Management	**0,97**	1578,45 (4-192) 0,000	0,30 (0,000)
Empathy	1,00	n.s. (5-191) n.s.	0.23 (n.s.)

n.s. = not significant

As for the hierarchy obtained in this analysis, it is the *Automotivation* variable that best explains *Emotional Intelligence*, with a coefficient of 0.77 (p = 0.000). This variable alone accounts for 60% of the explanatory value of the dependent variable. Next, the ability to *Manage Relationships in Groups* contributes a value of 0 = 0.46 (p = 0.000) to *Emotional Intelligence*. The *Self-awareness* variable predicts the dependent variable with a certain coefficient of 0.39 (p = 0.000). Finally, *Emotional Management* predicts the variable selected as dependent with a value of 0 = 0.30 and a significance level of 0.000.

Given their statistical significance, the results show that the selected variables explain, or predict, 97% of the overall variance of the dependent variable.

Chapter 5

5 - THE EMOTIONAL INTELLIGENCE OF THE NURSES STUDIED

In the critical analysis of the data obtained from the sample of nurses. We have taken into account the authors who have already looked into the matter, as well as other studies carried out, in this and other populations, which have studied emotional intelligence (EI) or EI abilities, not forgetting the theoretical framework explained in the first part of this work, as well as the theoretical construct that supports it. We also intend to compare the results obtained in this sample with other data collected from other populations, namely those resulting from the application of the same instrument in Branco's (1999) study of teachers. For reasons of organization, the results are analysed according to the structure used in the previous chapter.

The sample

A sample of nurses at an EPE hospital was given a questionnaire that included the EVB - CIE (consisting of five sub-scales), with the aim of validating the instrument in this population and getting to know the profile of emotional intelligence (EI) skills, through the respondents' self-perception and represented by the frequency with which each of the situations/items occur to them.

Overall, we can consider that the nurses were very receptive to the study: 214 nurses answered the questionnaire, which corresponds to an adherence rate of 68.2%. Some of the reasons for the drop in response rates are due to the fact that some nurses were away on vacation, and others didn't fill in the questionnaire due to forgetfulness, overwork or even personal refusal.

The sample consisted of 214 nurses, 73.8% of whom were female and 26.2% male. 71% of the nurses were aged between 21 and 30 (mean 29.49 and SD = 7.22). This result reveals a considerably young sample, not yet *mature from* the point of view of acquiring a wide variety of personal and professional experiences.

Regarding the professional category of the nurses studied. 71.9% are level I nurses, 20.6% are graduates, 5.1% are specialist nurses and only 1.8% are head nurses. According to data presented by the Portuguese Nurses' Association (2004), the average age of Portuguese nurses is 36.8 years, and more than 60% of the individuals in this professional group are under 41 years old. At a national level, there are 35727 nurses and 8147 nurses, which corresponds to 81% and 19%, respectively, of the 43874 members actively registered with the Order of Nurses (Ordem dos Enfermeiros, 2004). In terms of professional category, 86% of nurses are generalists and/or graduates and there are 7% of nurses with the category of specialist nurse and 4% with the category of head nurse (Idem). So, in terms of the characteristics of this sample, we can consider that the data was very close to the national distribution. It also confirms that the nursing profession in this institution continues to be mainly represented by women.

The instrument

With regard to the second part of the questionnaire - EVB - CIE, we found a low number of responses to the *other* item. This may indicate that the subjects in this sample are better prepared to answer closed questions than open questions. In fact, we were able to see during our research that, in terms of data collection and processing, the majority of studies follow quantitative research methodologies.

After the factorial analysis of the main components, using the Varimax rotation method, 84 items were obtained which suggest a grouping into 17 factors relating to the five capacities of emotional intelligence. Although one of the main purposes of factor analysis is to reduce the number of variables into groups of smaller variables, losing as little information as possible (Almeida and Freire, 2000; Elliot et al., 2001), it can be seen that, in this study, of the 85 items in the five sub-scales of the **Veiga Branco Scale of Emotional Intelligence Capacities,** only one was excluded. This is due to the fact that the scale has already been refined since it was validated with teachers.

The application of this scale to a sample of nurses does not seem to show any significant conceptual differences from that of teachers, applied by Branco in 1999. Thus, we can consider that the theoretical model and the debugging previously carried out (by validating the scale with teachers) are in line and agree with the responses of nurses. One difference that can be seen in this study is that we obtained 17 factors for the five sub-scales, whereas Branco (1999) obtained 18 factors in his study with teachers, using the same instrument.

In terms of fidelity and according to Bowling (1994), the sub-scales (corresponding to abilities) have alpha values that are considered acceptable, i.e. Cronbach's alphas >0.60. The sub-scale with the lowest internal consistency is *Emotion Management* with a Cronbach's alpha = 0.69.

Self-awareness

The nurses in our sample perceive themselves to be, on average and as a rule, self-aware. Our sample perceived themselves to be less self-aware than the sample of teachers, so the latter perceived themselves to be at a frequent or very frequent level (Branco, 1999). However, the dimensions (factors/components) found are close to those validated for teachers.

In the correlational analysis, self-awareness correlates moderately with the skills of Emotion Management and Self-Motivation. In a study of teachers, self-awareness showed a strong, significant and positive correlation with self-motivation (Branco, 1999).

The exploratory analysis of this ability revealed four factors. The same happened in the study on teachers (1999). These factors, according to the sample's self-perception, seem to measure the following aspects of Self-awareness, as explained below.

Emotional instability - Factor 1

According to the data obtained, nurses rarely (with a strong tendency towards infrequent) show emotional instability or are manipulated by negative feelings. In other words, they rarely take on behaviors that affect their emotional balance in the face of negative situations or relationships.

Rational and relational changes - Factor 2

In the sample, we found that nurses infrequently perceive themselves as having altered their thinking or their relationships. They infrequently perceive changes in their relational behavior and their capacity for mental attention in the face of unpleasant feelings.

Positive perception of yourself as a person - Factor 3

Of the nurses surveyed, it is the younger nurses (aged <40) who have the least frequent self-perception. Older nurses recognize that they tend to act as more positive, rational, observant, flexible and autonomous people. It is noteworthy that, in a study with teachers, Branco (1999) obtained exactly the same grouping of items.

Perception of the occurrence of emotional phenomena - Factor 4

In this context, it is also younger nurses who are less likely to perceive emotional phenomena in their lives. Nurses aged 40 or over feel, on average more often, that they are able to become aware of and identify their emotions, and are able to verbalize them and even push them away when they are negative emotions.

On average, the subjects in our sample self-perceived the occurrence of emotional phenomena as frequent. The same was found in the sample of teachers, with a tendency towards very frequent (Branco, 1999).

In this factor, we also obtained a grouping of items identical to that found in the study with teachers (Branco, 1999).

Emotion management

The average of the nurses surveyed perceived managing their emotions as infrequent, with a tendency towards the norm. In the sample of teachers studied by Branco (1999), there were better frequencies, with the latter placing their attributions at as a rule and frequently.

This ability correlates moderately with self-awareness and self-motivation. In Branco's study (1999, p.93), the researcher also detected "acceptable consistency" between emotion management and the other abilities.

In this capacity, five factors were obtained - exactly the same number as that found by Branco (1999) for teachers. The sample grouped them as follows.

Negative adaptation (intrusion, explosion) - Factor 5

Nurses, on average, rarely (with a strong tendency towards infrequently) perceive themselves to have intrusion or outburst styles of adaptation, i.e. they rarely isolate themselves or use objects, people or situations as targets for their anger in situations of anxiety or negative mood. In the study with teachers, the same grouping of items was obtained. However, they obtained higher frequencies, at the level of infrequent and as a rule (Branco, 1999).

Control using reason - Factor 6

Older nurses generally have greater control over using reason in situations of anger or rage compared to younger nurses. This means that older nurses (>40 years) try to reason without judgment, by examining, reassessing the situation and moving on to positive thoughts.

Escape and loneliness - Factor 7

As a rule, nurses self-perceive that, when faced with negative emotional situations, they tend to seek distraction or prefer to be alone, away from provocation. We highlight the fact that, in a study with teachers, Branco (1999) obtained exactly the same grouping of items, as well as an identical frequency of perception of the phenomenon.

Anxious, reactive feelings - Factor 8

The sample usually shows feelings of anxiety and reaction. In other words, when faced with unpleasant emotional situations, they usually feel anguish and worry, but in order to deal with them, they either think about them or divert their attention away from these emotions. Branco (1999), in a study of teachers, obtained a grouping of items similar to that found in this sample.

There is data pointing to the fact that, in general, women are more prone to mood disorders (Paúl and Fonseca, 2001). This was not confirmed in the sample of nurses studied.

Control by physical activity - Factor 9

Nurses, on average, infrequently resort to physical activity or sports for their emotional control. However, the data suggests that nurses use this strategy more than women nurses.

Automotive

The nurses in the sample perceive themselves, on average, as infrequently self-motivated, which is a somewhat worrying indicator to take into account when devising management strategies for this professional group. In the sample of teachers, Branco (1999) obtained higher temporal attributions - in the order of usually and often. This suggests that nurses perceive themselves as less self-motivated than teachers.

Of all the EI abilities, this is the one with the strongest and most significantly positive correlation with overall Emotional Intelligence, and the one that is most explanatory of Emotional Intelligence. In relation to the other abilities, self-motivation has moderate and positive correlations with self-awareness and emotion management.

In this capacity, we forced the items into three factors because two of the factors (1 and 3) tended to be grouped together. This ability was the one with the most variation compared to the validation with teachers carried out by Branco (1999), in which four factors associating the items of the self-motivation sub-scale were obtained. The following factors were obtained.

Illiterate, insecure and dependent - Factor 10

Rarely (with a tendency towards infrequent) do the nurses in the sample recognize themselves as insecure or dependent, not allowing themselves to be invaded by self-pity, pessimism or humiliation. However, younger nurses perceive themselves to be significantly more insecure and dependent than older nurses in situations of personal rejection (socially or professionally). In the case of teachers, this factor is often and usually present (Branco, 1999).

Literates use emotional energy - Factor 11

As a rule, the average of the sample perceives themselves as literate in the use of emotional energy, i.e. they feel they have sufficient ability to face problems, act after thinking and find a mitigating attitude to negative situations in their work. We highlight the fact that younger nurses perceive themselves as less skilled in the use of emotional energy than older nurses. The same perception is seen in the sample of teachers (Branco, 1999), with a tendency to frequent.

"State of flow" in activity (assets) - Factor 12

Nurses, on average, when performing a task or professional activity, infrequently feel in a state of activity in which they lose track of time and space, become absorbed in their surroundings or experience sensations of pleasure (personal enjoyment). The same perception was found in the sample of teachers (Branco, 1999).

According to Goleman (2000), men show greater self-confidence and optimism, adapt more easily and withstand stress better.

This data was not verified in the sample of nurses presented.

Empathy

The exploratory factorial analysis of the main components extracted three factors or main components of this ability. In this sub-scale, we highlight the fact that we obtained exactly the same number of factors, as well as the same items in each factor, as those found in the validation of the instrument in teachers (Branco, 1999).

The subjects in the sample perceive themselves, on average, as normally empathetic (with a tendency towards frequent), and age has a significant influence on this ability. Younger nurses perceived themselves as less empathetic than older ones. The sample of teachers (Branco, 1999) showed precisely the opposite. These self-perceived empathy at the frequent and very frequent levels, but younger teachers perceived themselves as more empathetic than older ones.

In nurses, the ability to empathize is moderately related to managing relationships in groups, with the highest inter-capacity correlation of all. In the study of teachers carried out by Branco (1999), this relationship was not found, suggesting that there is no consistent relationship between empathy and self-awareness and emotion management skills.

In terms of social awareness, empathy is the basis on which the team builds relationships with the rest of the organization (Goleman, Boyatzis and McKee, 2002). As such, empathy is an extremely important skill for the professional and therapeutic relationships that nurses establish. According to Goleman (2003), the skill of empathy emerges from self-awareness, but the results do not confirm this relationship, since, according to the self-perception of the sample of nurses, there is only a weak relationship between these two skills, even the weakest of all. The same was true of the study by Branco (2004b), in which the results did not confirm dependence or a consistent relationship between these two constructs, or between empathy and the other skills.

With regard to the predictive value of nurses' EI, empathy does not reach statistically significant levels, and is the only EI ability that has no explanatory power for Emotional Intelligence in this sample. However, in our sample, empathy is the ability that shows the strongest inter-skill relationship with Group Relationship Management.

Communication is a key aspect of the therapeutic relationship. It is essential to establish a true nurse-user dialog, based on empathy, in order to identify beliefs, motivations, difficulties and support that can promote the success of the care provided. Daniel (1983) states that empathy is "one of the inseparable principles of the ability to understand at the therapeutic level" (p.48) which, when developed and applied as a skill, leads to professional growth and a better quality of nursing care. On the other hand, Jesus (2004) points out that, although it may be suggested that high levels of EI favor better professional performance, the presence of high levels of empathy can lead to excessive identification with the patient, thus damaging the therapeutic relationship itself.

Although Goleman's (2000) studies have shown that, on average, women are more aware of emotions, show more empathy and are more competent in interpersonal relationships than men. This was not the case in our sample.

Values expression (verbal and non-verbal) - Factor 13

The sample normally values (with a considerable tendency to frequent) verbal and non-verbal expression in their relationships, i.e. they *usually value* gestures, voice, gaze and the consistency between words and body attitude. The same perception was found in the sample of teachers (Branco, 1999).

Relational harmony - Factor 14

The nurses in the sample usually (and often) experience harmony in their relationships with others (personal, family and professional). Thus, nurses generally feel in tune with the feelings of others and decode non-verbal channels. However, the data suggests statistically significant differences between age and this factor, with younger nurses being less able to establish relational attunement than nurses aged 40 or over.

The sample of teachers studied by Branco (1999) showed a greater perception of relational harmony, in the range of frequent and very frequent.

Serene attitude in conflict situations - Factor 15

On average, nurses usually (with a tendency towards frequently) display calm attitudes in conflict situations, using calmness to listen when faced with the instability of others. Teachers (Branco, 1999) self-perceived themselves in this factor at the frequent and very frequent level.

It is noteworthy that nurses working in *chronic* services are more calm and serene when faced with conflict situations than nurses working in *acute* services. Perhaps this result is due to the fact that the latter have more opportunity to get to know the people they work with (users, users' families, professionals, among others) more deeply than nurses in *acute* services.

Relationship management in groups

In this capacity, and by previously defining the number of factors we wanted to obtain for the confirmatory factorial analysis, two main components were obtained. Thus, the factors that emerged from this factorial solution were the same (in number and grouping of items) as those that emerged from the study on teachers (Branco, 1999).

As highlighted above, the ability to empathize is moderately related to the ability to manage relationships in groups, and these have the highest inter-capacity correlation of all.

On average, nurses *usually see themselves* as being able to manage relationships. However, it is the younger nurses who perceive themselves as having greater difficulty in managing relationships than the older nurses. In the same capacity, the sample of teachers studied by Branco (1999) showed lower frequencies - infrequent and as a rule. As well as being a considerably young sample, the vast majority of nurses do not have people in their care (71%), a fact which may influence the difficulties of younger individuals in managing relationships in groups, as they have not been faced with managing their family group.

In our sample, with regard to academic qualifications, we also found quite significant statistical differences, with the result that graduate nurses perceive themselves as more capable in this capacity than nurses with a bachelor's degree.

Another significant finding is that there are statistically significant differences between this ability and the type of service. Nurses working in *chronic* services manage relationships better than those working in *acute* services. According to Daniel (1983), nursing professionals need to be efficient in the performance of their work, which includes interpersonal relationships as a therapeutic process involving the patient and the family, with the aim of achieving a higher quality of nursing care.

Emotional perception and synchronism - Factor 16

Regarding the emotional perception and synchronism of the relationships they establish with other people (personally, socially or professionally), the sample perceives themselves, on average, with a frequency of per norm. In other words, nurses feel that they are usually able to pick up on the feelings of others, adjust to them and act in a way that influences them. In the sample of teachers (Branco, 1999), they showed less emotional perception and synchronism, with a frequency of rarely and infrequently.

In this factor, the data suggests that graduate nurses have a greater capacity to perceive their emotions and synchrony than nurses with a bachelor's degree.

Nurses under the age of 40 are also less emotionally aware and less in sync with others than older nurses, so there are statistically significant differences between the age of nurses and the factor of managing relationships in groups.

Personal and relational stability - Factor 17

On average, the nurses in the sample perceive themselves as having personal and relational stability with a frequency of *usually* (with a strong tendency towards often), i.e. they feel that they usually have stable personal relationships, with control over their own feelings. The same perception was confirmed in the sample of teachers (Branco, 1999).

In this sample, it was the younger nurses who showed less personal and relational stability than the older ones, with statistically significant differences between this factor and age.

There were also statistically significant differences between the factor and the type of service. Nurses who work predominantly in *acute* services are less likely to self-perceive personal and relational stability than nurses in *chronic* services. These findings are reinforced by the data found in the study with doctors and nurses in the emergency department, in which younger individuals had higher *Sensation Seeking* values, i.e. they are people with low dopamine production who seek out risky activities (physical or psychological) to stimulate and motivate themselves (Pinho, 1994, cited by Gandum and Pedro, 2005).

With regard to academic qualifications, the data suggests that nurses with a bachelor's degree perceive themselves as having greater personal and relational stability than those with a bachelor's degree.

Emotional Intelligence

On average, and according to their self-perception, nurses consider themselves to be emotionally intelligent infrequently (with a strong tendency towards normally). In a study of teachers (Branco, 1999), they showed frequencies of *usually* and *often*, i.e. they considered themselves slightly more competent than the nurses under study.

With regard to the type of service in which the nurses surveyed work, the data suggests that there are statistically significant differences with regard to Emotional Intelligence. Thus, nurses working in the type of service known as *chronic* self-perceived themselves as emotionally intelligent more often than nurses working in services known as *acute*.

Pinho's 1994 study also concluded that there is a significant relationship between personality traits and the tasks these professionals perform. In other words, emergency room nurses are more *Sensation Seeking* than their colleagues on the wards (Pinho, 1994, cited by Gandum and Pedro, 2005). In the study by Jesus (2004), nurses whose clinical decision-making processes were more methodical, organized and closer to the users had higher levels of SI.

In terms of global EI, no statistically significant differences were found with the other characterization variables selected, including gender. Despite the slight differences found in Goleman's studies, in general, there are many similarities between men and women (Goleman, 2000). In fact, in the generic results for both sexes, the weaknesses and strengths offset each other, so that in terms of total EI, the data does not suggest that there are any differences between the sexes.

Nurses, as health professionals, are agents who promote healthy behaviors, which help in the process of adapting to illness and/or life problems. This being the case, and given the reality found in this population, the question is asked:

> *How can nurses be efficient in the care they provide* if they are not the *first to possess - usually or often - emotional competence?*

According to Goleman (2000), emotional competence is based on Emotional Intelligence, which is observable, for example, in professional practice. Therefore, the data found in this sample of nurses points to a positive and significant correlation between EI skills and between these and overall EI. This can be supported by the fact that psychosocial variables rarely exceed Pearson's r values of 0.50 (Polit and Hungler, 1995). In this way, the constructs were validated by the sample with significant correlations for an overall significance level of p <0.01. However, the results show a different correlation between skills and EI, which could be a relevant factor when defining nurses' training strategies.

The highest correlations were found between overall Emotional Intelligence and the skills of self-awareness, emotion management and self-motivation. There were moderate correlations with empathy and managing relationships in groups.

In the sample, the five sub-scales (which measure the dimensions/capabilities of EI) are related to overall Emotional Intelligence. However, the theoretical assumptions are validated in a different way in the sample of nurses studied. The EI abilities show the strongest positive correlations with: 1st - Self-motivation, 2nd - Managing emotions, 3rd - Self-awareness, 4th - Managing relationships in groups and 5th - Empathy - suggesting that this ability has the least influence on nurses' emotional intelligence. Also in the study with teachers (Branco, 1999), the ability to empathize "(...) has the least influence on the variability of emotional competence (...)" (p.96).

With regard to the validation of the instrument based on the sample's responses and the respective inter-variable correlational level, we can consider, from an overall perspective, that all the factors, abilities and overall Emotional Intelligence show positive and significant correlations, but not as recommended in Goleman's theoretical model (2000, 2003). Overall, the sample shows mostly attitudes and behaviors that, using Damasio's (1995) words, emerge from negative body states.

The cluster image that identifies the EI profile of these nurses is represented by two types of skills - intrapersonal and interpersonal (Goleman, 2000, 2003). The first type is made up of three abilities that represent skills at the subject's intrapersonal level - Self-motivation, Emotion Management followed by Self-awareness. The second type of skills refers to interpersonal skills, as they represent the subject's social interaction with contexts, and is made up of Factor 16 - Emotional Perception and Synchronism - followed by the skills of Relationship Management in Groups and Empathy.

The theoretical perspective defended by Goleman (2000, 2003) that EI emerges from the level of Self-Awareness is not, here, configured by the sample. According to the perception of this sample, the most influential ability in the variability of this EI profile is Self-motivation, considered by Goleman (2000, 2003) to be the third ability, followed by Emotion Management. The third correlation is Self-awareness. It can be seen that there is an inversion of semantic meaning between the construct and the sample's perception of the third and first EI capability.

If, for Goleman, obtaining a good level of EI comes from the ability to scrutinize the occurrence of emotions in one's own body and, based on this skill, be able to manage the emotional phenomena perceived and, after this management, configure attitudinal aspects inherent to Self-motivation, for the sample it is precisely Self-motivation that ensures the level of variability of their EI. Regardless of the correlation between Emotional Intelligence and Self-Awareness, it is now important to understand how the sample configures the exercise of this capacity.

Does this capacity include the attitudes and behaviors envisioned by the theoretical construct? This is not always the case. According to the sample's perception, self-motivation is achieved in nursing *practice,* but not through emotional tendencies that facilitate the fulfillment of their work objectives, based on optimism, the will to succeed, commitment and initiative (Goleman, 2000, 2003). Rather, the interpretation of the results suggests that self-motivation is related to the phenomena of insecurity and dependence (F10), negative adaptation (F5) and emotional instability (F1). Although Goleman translates this ability into positive attributions of internality, this population of nurses perceives their self-motivation and seems to be able to obtain energy for their work through not very proficient states of mind. Apart from these, they only achieve this (self-motivation) through a positive factor which concerns their perception of states of "flow" in activity (F12), losing track of time and space and feeling pleasure in the activities they carry out.

Considering that nursing *practice has* two essential pillars - the therapeutic relationship and the technical-scientific component - this Self-Motivation profile not only suggests that this professional population gives more importance to technicality to the detriment of the therapeutic relationship - to which several theorists allude and the training *curricula* present - but furthermore, and as a consequence, it seems that it is through this technical component that these nurses mobilize their motivational energy.

Why does this sample shape their Aitionioiivaeao in this way? Does this sense of professional efficacy emerge from a personal perspective on the meaning of their profession, or is it anchored in an emergence to meet the institutional needs/demands that nurses urgently need to meet, given the behaviors and attitudes reflected in the factors that make up Self-Motivation - F10, F12, F5 and F1? If the characterization variables (e.g. liking the workplace; professional fulfilment; ideas being listened to and put into practice; enjoying being a nurse; experiencing levels of success in the care provided; among others) do not show a negative feeling of being in the profession, how does self-motivation emerge from such negative states of mind (Damásio, 1995)?

With regard to the Emotion Management ability, this population of nurses manages their emotions from the same perspective as the previous ability, i.e. emerging from "negative body states" (Damásio, 19995). This ability repeats the F5 and F10 factors present in Self-motivation and Self-awareness (as they show significant correlations in both abilities), which demonstrate how these nurses manage their own internal states, impulses and resources (Goleman, 2000, 2003).

The answers obtained from the sample associate emotion management mechanisms based on: Negative adaptation (F5), Anxious and reactive feelings (F8), Escape and loneliness (F7), Illiteracy with insecurity and dependence (F10) and Control through physical activity (F9). In the light of Goleman's model, Emotion Management competence is achieved through self-mastery, inspiring confidence, adapting to change and being open to new ideas and information (Goleman, 2000, 2003), criteria which are not met by these nurses.

Self-awareness, the last ability in the intrapersonal competencies in this sample, is made up of the same type of grouping as the previous abilities, with behaviors and attitudes catalogued as negative. In this ability, the sample repeats three factors from Self-motivation and two from Lunch Management, thus maintaining the negative pattern of the previous abilities.

The way in which these nurses know their internal states, preferences, resources and intuitions (Goleman, 2000, 2003), is through: Emotional instability (F1), Rational and relational changes (F2), Negative adaptation (F5) and Illiteracy with insecurity and dependence (F10). The only factor that is in line with Goleman's definition is F4 - Perception of the occurrence of emotional phenomena - through which these nurses are able to get to know themselves. These results do not confirm what Goleman advocates for a person who has the capacity for Self-Awareness. According to the author (2000, 2003), mastering this ability implies recognizing one's own emotions, strengths and limitations, with self-confidence in one's abilities and self-worth.

The data obtained in this first unit of analysis - intrapersonal skills - can be explained by the fact that their working situation has not yet been defined. These nurses, most of whom are young, have not yet stabilized their careers, nor have they defined their position and status among their peers.

With regard to the interpersonal profile, the sample considers the skills of Emotional Perception and Synchronism (F16) to be a priority over Relationship Management in Groups and Empathy. However, this factor includes and overlaps the factorial correlations of the two subsequent skills. It is this phenomenon that translates the new contextual evidence of the sample, regardless of the semantic and correlational value of each of these three skills.

Emotional perception and synchronization (F16) emerges as one of the skills that make up the interpersonal competences of the EI of this sample. The nurses studied perceive their emotions and synchronize with others through: Valuing verbal and non-verbal expression (F13), Relational attunement (F14), Literate use of emotional energy (F11) and Personal and relational stability (F17).

The first skill in this group of competencies is Managing Relationships in Groups. The nurses studied perceive the ability to induce favorable responses in others, associating factors that are in line with what Goleman advocates. The author considers the skills - effective persuasion, open listening, conflict resolution, leadership, initiating and managing change, creating bonds and working as a team towards common goals - to be fundamental to the competence of managing Relationships in Groups (Goleman, 2000, 2003). In the sample studied, the nurses revealed this skill through: Emotional perception and synchronism (F16), Personal and relational stability (F17), Literate using emotional energy (F11), Valuing verbal and non-verbal expression (F13), Relational attunement (F14), Positive perception of self as a person (F3), Serene attitude in conflict situations (F15) and Control using reason (F6). In this way, the sample's responses are in line with the theoretical model that underpins this research.

The second skill that makes up this type of interpersonal/social competence is Empathy. According to the theoretical construct, this ability implies being aware of the feelings and needs of others, adopting attitudes of: understanding others, developing the skills of those with whom they relate, meeting the needs of clients/users, enhancing diversity and being able to read the emotions and power relations of a group (Goleman, 2000, 2003). Although Empathy did not prove to be predictive of Emotional Intelligence (through *hierarchical multiple regression*), this ability does associate - with moderate and high positive correlations - the factors: Values verbal and non-verbal expression (F13), Relational attunement (F14), Emotional perception and synchronism (F16), Positive attitude in conflict situations (F15), Literates using emotional energy (F11), Positive perception of oneself as a person (F3) and Perception of the occurrence of emotional phenomena (F4).

After describing this last set of skills, three facts become relevant:

Firstly, all of the variables (behavioral and attitudinal) that make it up have a positive emotional value, from which we can deduce that nurses only configure their positive skills in interaction with others and not with themselves. It is precisely this aspect that may provide some justification for the negative factors - mentioned above when explaining the intrapersonal skills of the sample. If the configurations of Self-motivation were anchored in technicality and Lunch Management in negative adaptation and avoidance, and Self-awareness lacked a positive perception of oneself as a person (F3) - a fact of the utmost importance - it is now in the contextual interaction with the other that the therapeutic relationship re-emerges, apparently omitted from these intrapersonal dimensions. This could mean that the phenomena of a positive emotional nature are not omitted in the nursing work context, but are omitted in the subject's interaction with him/herself, while in the relationship with the other they are intact. The vast majority of these nurses believe that the interpersonal relationship with users is very important for the success of the care they provide, and that their emotional stability contributes to the interpersonal relationship. This finding explains the positive sense that the nurses studied attribute to relational aspects, since the relationship itself with people is very, or quite, important for their emotional stability. It seems to be in this *interactive game* that nurses find their positive emotional energy.

Secondly, in this grouping of two skills and one factor, some factors (F11, F13 and F14) which relate to positive emotional phenomena are systematically repeated.

Thirdly, it should be noted that only the skills - Group Relationship Management and Empathy - are part of the positive perception of oneself as a person (F3). In other words, only when nurses manage group relationships (peers, users and students) and experience empathetic relationships do they have a positive perception of themselves. Goleman (2000, 2003) considers positive self-perception to be the essential energy for mobilizing empathic capacity - which, curiously, is not perceived by the sample as predictive of EI and, therefore, for interaction in human contexts and interpersonal relationships. At this point, the contradiction between the theoretical construct and the sample's perception values is worrying.

Emotional Perception and Synchronism (F16), when selected by the sample for its EI profile, illustrates a curious phenomenon. Apparently, only when it is correlated with the behaviors and attitudes of Managing Relationships in Groups and Empathy, does it select exactly the most positive emotional valuation factors among some of the abilities that, in a factorial analysis of the abilities alone, make up this profile - extracting F11 from Self-motivation; extracting factors F11, F13 and F14 from Empathy; and integrating F17 which, in a factor analysis, integrates and Managing Relationships in Groups. In other words, nurses selectively build a *new* ability which seems to act as a bridge between the subject's intrapersonal and interpersonal skills.

Using hierarchical regression analysis (Stepwise method), we can confirm that the ability with the best predictive value for Emotional Intelligence is self-motivation. This variable alone accounts for 60% of the explanatory value of nurses' EI. Next comes the ability to manage relationships in groups, then self-awareness and, lastly, managing emotions. The analysis selected the four variables mentioned, excluding empathy and gender, as they did not reach statistical significance. Given their statistical significance, the results show that the selected variables explain or predict 97% of the overall variance of the dependent variable (Emotional Intelligence), i.e. the analysis in this sample seems to partially validate the theoretical construct, but in a different way. In the study of teachers (Branco, 1999), the five subscales are predictive of emotional intelligence, and none of the EI abilities were eliminated.

Cadman and Brewer (2001) state that EI includes self-control, enthusiasm, persistence, the ability to motivate oneself and altruism. At the heart of altruism lies empathy or the ability to read emotion in others, which in turn is the basis of the therapeutic relationship. If this capacity is limited, or doesn't exist at all, and if there is no capacity to feel the other person's needs or suffering, then there can be no therapeutic relationship. Health professionals have the task of establishing helping relationships and must be able to respond to patients' emotions, and it is difficult to understand how this can happen if these same professionals are unable to create an empathetic relationship (Reynolds and Scott 2000, cited by Cadman and Brewer, 2001). Bellack (1999) also states that the ability to empathize - one of the social skills - highlights the importance of being able to show interest and concern for others, recognize and respond to the patient's needs, value diversity, have political awareness, know how to listen and communicate, influence and inspire others; manage change, resolve conflicts, cooperate and collaborate with others to achieve common goals. Thus, this study confirms the results of previous research which indicates that empathy is not the attitude taken by the majority of professionals, including nurses, who are unable to demonstrate high levels of empathy (Williams, 1992, Sloane, 1993, Baillie 1995, 1996, cited by Cadman and Brewer, 2001). This reality is compromising, as Reynolds and Scott (2000, cited by Cadman and Brewer, 2001) state that the various pieces of evidence collected indicate a direct relationship between the levels of empathy demonstrated by nurses and positive patient outcomes. Given these results, we wonder: *If nursing curricula are concerned with developing these skills in students, why does empathy not predict the EI of the nurses studied?*

At a time when there is so much discussion about higher education reforms in the light of the Bologna Process, any kind of reform in nursing education should achieve more than the usual minor changes to *curricula*. Overall, we believe that nursing curricula are doing a very good job of educating students and preparing them for the cognitive and technical aspects of their work. What may be lacking in the way future nursing professionals are prepared are the emotional skills that the complexity of our health system demands and that American health managers have already called for (Bellack, 1999). Analysis of the results of the application of the Empathy sub-scale suggests that this ability is being sidelined, perhaps because of the imperatives inherent in the current context of professional practice, as mentioned above.

The fact that, in this sample, age influenced eight factors and two EI skills (empathy and managing relationships in groups) can be explained with the help of Goleman (2000). The author states that, unlike IQ, which changes little after adolescence, EI is assimilated and continues to develop throughout life, as we learn from our experiences. The author uses an elucidating word to define this growth in EI - "maturity" (Idem, p.15). This is important because, according to Sprinthall (1980, cited by Almeida e Silva, 1993, In Branco, 2004b), success in life is more related to psychological maturity than to school results.

When we talk about age, we inevitably associate it with length of service. Therefore, an older nurse is also a nurse who has worked for longer. With regard to this sample, we can say that older age and more work experience are synonymous with greater self-perception:

- Empathy and relationship management in groups;
- Positive perception of oneself as a person;
- Occurrence of emotional phenomena;
- Control using reason;
- Security and independence;
- Using emotional energy to self-motivate;
- Relational attunement;
- Emotional perception and synchronization with others;
- Personal and relationship stability.

Despite the fact that 60 nurses (28.04%) were immigrants, there were no statistically significant differences between them and Portuguese nurses in terms of factors, abilities and Emotional Intelligence.
The same was true of the postgraduate training variable.

PART III

APPLIED EMOTIONAL COMPETENCE

In view of the results obtained in our and other studies, some considerations deserve to be taken into account in order to sensitize nursing managers and educators to reflect on how to promote and develop the emotional competence of nursing professionals. We want to believe that knowledge of nurses' EI skills can be used as a contribution to the management, training, recruitment and performance evaluation of these professionals.

Emotional intelligence (EI) skills can be learned and developed throughout life (Goleman, 2000, 2003). The training and emotional education of nurses is a way of promoting a good working climate and, in turn, optimizing the quality of health care provided by these professionals. Therefore, in the following pages, emphasis will be placed on the interest of emotional intelligence skills for the professional nursing group.

Chapter 6

6 - IN HEALTHCARE ORGANIZATIONS

The Order of Nurses (2001, p.5) states in one of its publications that "it is up to health institutions to adapt the resources and create the structures that facilitate quality professional practice". In this sense, health institutions must provide the conditions that facilitate nurses' professional and even personal development. Schilling (1996, cited by Salovey, Mayer and Caruso, 2002) recommends self-help units, where people learn (often through group dynamics) to control their feelings when making decisions, manage stress, increase personal responsibility and self-concept, develop empathy, communicate and resolve conflicts.

Viriginia Ladd (cited by Costa, 2005), a member of the AIOP Council[1] and a sufferer of a serious chronic illness, says that good relationships between patients and the health professionals who care for them are based on mutual respect, trust and good communication. It is easy to understand that, in this way, more advantageous results are achieved for both patients and health professionals, in terms of stricter compliance with therapies and greater satisfaction with the quality of care provided.

In a study carried out by Jesus (2004), in which nursing clinical decision-making patterns were studied, three skills inherent to this process were compared - emotional intelligence (EI),

---

[1] The International Alliance of Patients' Organizations (IAOP) is the only worldwide alliance representing patients of all nationalities suffering from any disease. AIOP believes that, throughout the world, patients should be the center of health care (Viriginia Ladd, cited by Costa, 2005).

critical thinking and creative thinking. Thus, the author identified two patterns of clinical decision-making in the nurses studied. Pattern A, with higher mean and median *scores* in the overall EI test used, is "indicative of a care process that is methodical, personalized, intimate with the patient, rigorous, attentive, helpful, empathetic, reflective, based on aspects of the helping relationship, engaging and compassionate" (Jesus, 2004, p.359). Pattern B, with lower average and median *scores* in the overall EI test used, is "indicative of a more functional care process, centred on activity, more superficial and reductionist, less organized, with a more instrumental, less communicative and less human relationship with the patient" (Idem, p.359-360).

According to Martins et al. (2003), while users are looking for more humane and quality care, the susceptibility of the National Health Service (SNS) to financial and commercial imperatives hinders the development of care with these characteristics. He goes on to say that emotionally competent care is economically tangible and makes citizens (NHS clients) more satisfied with the professionals and institutions that assist them. These conclusions undoubtedly help us to understand how EI can make an important contribution to the quality of care processes, in any organization or service.

In the United States, many employers claim that nursing schools are graduating students who lack the necessary skills to adapt successfully to the world of work (Bellack, 1999). This author reinforces that both cognitive intelligence and proficiency in nursing practice are necessary and are basic requirements for starting nursing practice. But despite these, and according to Goleman (2003, cited by Bellack, 1999), a third skill in the world of work, emotional intelligence, is fundamental and essential for proper work performance, regardless of the type of task or work environment.

In this way, we believe that nursing professionals in a hospital unit should be distributed according to their EI competencies and skills, so that they can achieve greater sensitivity and adaptation to the characteristics and typology of the patients they care for, in order to achieve the highest levels of client satisfaction. In this way, this study can provide a basis for defining an instrument to support the recruitment/selection of new nurses in a health institution, as well as for the reassignment of professionals by service according to their emotional intelligence skills. Goleman (2000) points out that emotional intelligence skills are synergistic and compatible with cognitive ones, so the best professionals possess both. The more complex the job - as is the case in the nursing profession - the more important the role of EI. A lack of these skills can hinder the normal development of any experience or intellect.

The application of the EVB-CIE in this sample of nurses differs from that of teachers, applied by Branco in 1999. We therefore believe that the emotional education strategies to be adopted by management and training bodies should take into account the specificity of the data found, developing these emotional skills in nurses in an informed way.

Developing a good organizational *climate, in the* sense of getting to know it and improving it, means investing in an in-depth analysis of your employees. Ignoring this behavior, leaving it to each individual, boss or team, and creating a work spirit that is outside the organization's mission and vision, seems to us to be a highway to chaos.

6.1 - CONTRIBUTIONS TO MANAGEMENT

Possible interventions to develop EI can also be found in the workplace. These programs are of a much more advanced stage of development than those designed for the basic training of students and professionals (Goleman. 2000. 2003. Salovey. Mayer and Caruso. 2002). In addition. many of these EI programs. in the workplace. are sessions where relationships are trained. motivation for work. stress management and the resolution of existing conflicts in the organization (Idem).

Walsh and Walsh (1998) interestingly state that a patient may be very satisfied with the nursing care received, but not so satisfied with the meals provided at the hospital or the attitude of a member of staff. This is where the importance of processes to assess the characteristics and qualities of staff, in this case nurses, comes in, in order to introduce mechanisms to develop the skills needed to provide higher quality care.

At a meeting of health managers in the state of South Carolina, participants pointed out that recently graduated nurses enter the world of work with a diploma and credentials, but they lack certain skills such as common sense, work ethic, organizational skills, knowing when to call in another member of their team and an interest in continuing education (South Carolina Colleagues in Caring, 1998, cited by Bellack, 1999). This perception shouldn't extend too far from the Portuguese reality and it could be said that these are some of the skills that Goleman relates to EI, because, in fact, EI is clearly desirable and necessary in a profession as intensely based on relationships and service organization as nursing is.

According to Witt et al. (cited by Colell Brunet et al., 2004), in order to provide the best possible care for patients with advanced and terminal illnesses, as well as their families, specific training and emotional preparation is necessary. Colell Brunet et al. (2004) also report that, when we focus on the professional nursing group, there is no doubt that the skills of expressing, understanding and regulating emotions, as well as the capacity for perceived control, can be aspects that help us to cope with the stress generated by working with the illness and the terminally ill patient. Caring for a terminally ill patient (and their family) generates intense emotions in healthcare professionals. On the other hand, the emotional impact of working with death and suffering on a daily basis can hinder good professional practice. Limonero et al. (2004, cited by Colell Brunet et al., 2004) also point out that the ability to assess and distinguish between patients' emotional responses and to use this information as a guide for thoughts and actions can be important in re-establishing the nurse-patient relationship.

According to Elam (2000, cited by Colell Brunet et al., 2004), the effective handling of emotional responses can be an important dimension in helping nursing professionals to assess and overcome work-related stress. Although stress is usually considered *harmful* by many, there are some people who seem to need it. This is the case with some nurses and doctors who, despite the stressful environment they experience in hospital emergency departments, enjoy and want to work there. Pilots, air traffic controllers, police officers, firefighters and high-level sportsmen and women are also mentioned by Zuckerman (cited by Gandum and Pedro, 2005) as people who seek out stressful activities.

We found a contribution to clarifying this *paradox in* a study carried out by nurse Paula Pinho, in which the author applied the SSSV scale (Sensation Seeking Scale - developed and published in 1994 by Marvin Zuckerman, a specialist in these types of behavioral studies) to 100 doctors and nurses in Lisbon's emergency medical services. In order to understand the results of this study, two concepts need to be clarified. Firstly, *Sensation Seekers* are people with low production of dopamine (a neurotransmitter) who seek out risky activities (physical or psychological) in order to produce enough dopamine to function at normal levels, as an alternative to stimulants, It can also be called a kind of stress, "except that people with this kind of stress don't go into hysterics, because it's that very stress that motivates them to live" (Pinho, cited by Gandum and Pedro, 2005, p. 70).70). According to the author, the SSSV is an interval scale that measures four dimensions of the *Sensation Seeking* personality trait: risk-seeking adventure, experience-seeking, disinhibition and susceptibility to boredom. This study concluded that there is a relationship between personality traits and the tasks these professionals perform. Therefore, the author concluded, among other results, that:

- Emergency room doctors and nurses are more *Sensation Seeking* than their colleagues in the wards;
- Nurses are even more *Sensation Seeking* than doctors (perhaps due to the fact that nurses choose the emergency room as their workplace and doctors have a legal and curricular obligation to work 12 hours a week in the emergency room);
- Younger people have high *Sensation Seeking scores*.

Fornés et al. (2004) validated and found a factorial solution for the *Cuestionario de Hostigamiento Psicológico en el trabajo in* a sample of nursing professionals from the Balearic Islands. The study was based on the need to study professional harassment in this group, given that nurses are a group that has a number of difficulties in terms of professional autonomy and the social image of the profession due to historical dependence on the medical profession. This fact, although changing, makes it difficult (in certain contexts) to manage relationships with the multi-professional team, which affects their emotional balance.

In the results of the study *Implicación de la Inteligencia Emocional en Profesionales de Cuidados Paliativos,* Colell Brunet et al. (2004) obtained data showing that EI can have a beneficial effect when it comes to reducing the impact that death can have on healthcare professionals, specifically nurses, as they are the group that spends the most time with terminally ill patients. Tomás-Sábado (cited by Colell Brunet et al., 2004) points out that nurses who are frequently confronted with the death of their patients can face attitudes of rejection, doubt and insecurity, among other dysfunctions, due to the fact that they have to face their own fears in the face of death. It is clear that these attitudes hinder the provision of care in therapeutic or even palliative processes.

With this data, we asked ourselves two other questions:

How do nurses perceive their emotional capacities?

When faced with unfavorable situations (in life and at work), are nurses aware of their emotions and do they act accordingly?

It makes sense for us to study nurses' EI skills from the perspective of managing and training emotionally competent nurses. Providing nursing human resource managers with an instrument to facilitate knowledge of nurses' emotional competencies, adopting strategies to educate their employees emotionally, is yet another way of improving individual and team performance. According to Branco (2004b, p.49), "A person with high emotional competence is one who also has a high perception of what they can and cannot control". Therefore, this idea becomes essential in this study in the sense that, through each person's self-perception of their EI abilities, it will be possible to better understand how these interfere with professional performance, and how they can be used to improve professional processes and relationships.

According to Bellack (1999), managers at various levels of the hierarchy are responsible for their employees, as well as for the quality of care provided to users. They must therefore ensure that their employees acquire the social and personal skills to be able to use their technical and cognitive knowledge to the best of their ability. The researcher Vitello-Cicciu (2003) points out that successful operational managers (head nurses) and senior managers themselves create empathy with the members of their teams, fostering individual and group relationships, as well as recognizing the individual co-responsibilities of each team member who is part of the health organization. These same managers/leaders analyze the emotional side of issues and questions, anticipating people's reactions and creating programs that can assist teams with the emotional impact of issues related to their work. To do this requires certain characteristics, including the ability to identify emotions, to use emotions in the thinking process and to understand and analyze emotions, knowing how to deal with them in relation to oneself and others. Those who possess these abilities are emotionally intelligent individuals (Kerfoot, 1996, cited by Vitello-Cicciu, 2003).

The study of emotional skills and the recognition of their importance is a need that has been noted by several authors. A manager cannot ignore this fact, as the success of nurses' professional performance and, consequently, that of the entire team involved in providing health care to citizens, depends on this recognition (Bellack, 1999). According to Vitello-Cicciu (2003), nurse managers who are emotionally intelligent are role models in terms of their ability to manage their own emotions and, at the same time, manage their emotional responses towards their team members, patients and families.

6.1.1 - Leadership model

According to Dias (2005), head nurses are usually selected on the basis of their characteristics, administrative functions and knowledge. This author points out that there is usually no match between the type of leader behavior desired and the characteristics of the context in which they will perform their duties. On the other hand, Goleman, Boyatzis and McKee (2002, p.29) state that it is the leaders who determine the emotional pattern, and when the *official or formal leader* lacks credibility, people will look for emotional leadership from someone else they admire or respect. These authors also add that the actions of the boss/leader explain 50 to 70% of employees' feelings and moods in relation to the work environment and are therefore the most frequently cited reason for leaving a job - dissatisfaction with the boss.

The work environment has a very positive impact on professional performance and contributes greatly to the organization's results (Kelner, Rivers and O'Connell, 1994, Kozlowski and Doherty, 1989, Litwin and Stringer, 1968, cited by Cherniss, 2000, p.450). It's a *snowball* that begins, to a large extent, with the leader's EI skills. Thus, Benjamin Schneider (cited by Goleman, Boyatzis and McKee, 2002) discovered that employees' appreciation of the work environment was a good indicator for predicting the degree of customer satisfaction, which is synonymous with tangible results for the company.

Contrary to what usually appears, there are leaders in every position of an organization's hierarchy. Leadership is not only in the person who occupies the highest hierarchical position, but is spread across all individuals who, in one way or another, function as leaders of a group of followers (Goleman, Boyatzis and McKee, 2002).

The states of mind that the leader can transmit affect the group's results both positively and negatively, with the associated fact that "the greater the leader's ability to transmit emotions, the more intensely the emotions will spread" (Goleman, Boyatzis and McKee, 2002, p.31). The same authors also reinforce that great leadership is based on emotions, introducing a new concept, *Primal Leadership, in* which they state that leaders must conduct emotions correctly if they want to achieve positive effects on the strategy and success of their organizations. Although it is often invisible or ignored, the *primal* dimension of leadership consists of enhancing positive feelings in the people being led, creating *resonance*, i.e. increasing the intensity of positive feelings around them. The leader's emotional role is primal, that is, it comes first and at the same time is the most important, functioning as emotional guides for groups, directing the collective's emotions (Goleman, Boyatzis and McKee, 2002).

The old models of leadership were centered on the functions that the leader performed, not taking into account emotions or the personal dimension, and people were considered to be replaceable handles. Today, this type of leadership is increasingly in crisis (Goleman, Boyatzis and McKee, 2002). These authors say that "resonant leaders are shaking up the old type of leadership, which was shaped in the image of captains of industry, those old-fashioned figures of authority and leadership from the top, who led basically by virtue of positions of power" (Idem, p.267).

In the context of hospital nursing practice, the main player in team dynamics is the head nurse (Dias, 2005). According to this author, the head nurse is a fundamental element, as a manager of leadership and motivation of his/her employees, for the effective functioning of work groups (Dias, 2005). However, the best leaders are not only leaders by virtue of the position they occupy, but rather because they excel in the art of relationships, a skill that is increasingly indispensable due to the changes in organizational environments (Goleman, Boyatzis and McKee, 2002).

In a leadership model, four major fundamental domains of EI are listed: self-awareness; self-management; social awareness and relationship management (Goleman, Boyatzis and McKee, 2002). These researchers also break down certain competencies within each of the groups that form the basis of primal leadership. Each of these competencies provides a set of skills necessary for resonant leadership, which not only has an impact on the organization or company, but also on personal and family life.

6.1.1.1 - Leadership styles

Presenting a new model for cataloging types of leadership, Goleman, Boyatzis and McKee (2002) associate the understanding of EI competencies with each leadership style and establish the causal relationship between each style and the effects on the work climate and professional performance. In this context, the authors state that in order to be a good leader, you have to be skilled enough to change your style according to the needs and circumstances that arise and that, depending on the hierarchical level in the organization, certain leadership styles work better. Four of these styles resonate and lead to improvements in performance: the *visionary*, the *counselor*, the *relational* and the *democratic.* The other two types - *pressurizing* and *directive* - can be useful in special situations, but should be used carefully and in *small doses,* as they can create a very negative climate and, consequently, dissonance. The latter can interfere with employees' personal commitment if they are misused (Goleman, Boyatzis and McKee, 2002). These authors define the words *resonant* and *dissonant* using the roots of the words: *resonant* has its origin in *resonare,* which means to *resonate* or echo; dissonant means harsh or unpleasant sounds and designates a lack of harmony, which discourages people, exhausts them or drives them away, with repercussions at various levels - work, personal and family (Idem).

When it comes to leading teams, the motivational route can prove to be quite satisfactory in terms of its results. Goleman, Boyatzis and McKee (2002) state that effective leaders usually master at least one competency from each of the four fundamental areas of leadership competencies - self-awareness, self-management, social awareness and relationship management. However, they say they have never met a leader who has mastered all the EI competencies. What's more, they say that there is no single formula for effective leadership, so the best leaders can have very different personal styles and are, even the very effective ones, only strong in about half a dozen of these competencies. This proposal for emotion-based leadership is based on the EI skills described above (Goleman, 2000. 2003).
The emotionally intelligent leader captures emotions (sadness, joy, anguish, etc.) and expresses them to the group. If the leader doesn't use a good dose of feelings, he may be able to direct, but not lead. Even humour takes the group's emotional centers into a zone of positive activity, helping the group to avoid being submerged by negative emotions or discouragement and directing them towards solving the organization's problems (Goleman, Boyatzis and McKee, 2002).

In addition to leaders who use leadership styles with emotionally positive effects, those who use various styles depending on the situation and the need achieve clearly better results than other leaders. This is what Goleman, Boyatzis and McKee (2002, p.76) call "leading with class - the right style at the right time". Resonant leaders know when to be visionary, when to listen and when to give orders. They are insightful leaders who naturally nurture relationships, creating human synergies in harmonious groups. They make their employees loyal, because they care about their subordinates' careers and encourage people to give the best of themselves in pursuit of a mission that appeals to shared values (Idem). They also add that:

"Emotionally intelligent leaders do each of these things at the right time, in the right way and with the right people. This type of leadership generates a climate of enthusiasm and flexibility in which people are called upon to be innovative and give their best. (...) Leaders of this type are more values-driven, more flexible, more informal, more open and more frank (...)" (Goleman, Boyatzis and McKee, 2002, p.267-268).

6.1.1.2 - Effects of leadership on organizations

In their book, Goleman, Boyatzis and McKee (2002) give a surprising account of an example of emotional leadership. The protagonist of one of the cases was Mark Loehr, when his company was shaken by the deaths of countless employees and family members as a result of the September 11, 2001 attack on the twin towers in New York (Idem). This leader managed to create a positive resonance with his employees, providing a way of interpreting and making sense of the situation so that depression and crisis didn't set in, seriously damaging the organizational climate.

Another example, cited by Goleman, Boyatzis and McKee (2002), was what happened in the BBC news section, where the differences in manner and tone used by two different managers to broadcast the news of the section's closure were highlighted. One of the managers was almost assaulted, while the other was applauded. The first used hostility and antagonism; the second directed the group towards inspiring action and optimism. In this way, the two managers provoked two types of reactions in the workers. In the first case, negative feelings prevailed, the so-called dissonance; in the second case, they reacted positively, in other words, the leader generated resonance.

Returning to the work contexts of nurses, where the demands of the job on the level of emotions and empathy on the part of professionals is great, the resonance capacity of leaders becomes vital, enabling them to create work environments that are favorable to good professional performance and the optimization of results. In a study carried out by Dias (2005) on the style of leadership that allows the head nurse to optimize the effective performance of his/her employees, keeping them at the highest levels of motivation, it was concluded that the head nurse who maintains a high regard for the feelings and emotions of subordinate nurses is the one who proves to be the greatest facilitator of group interaction in order to achieve the stipulated objectives.

According to Goleman, Boyat/is and McKee (2002), even a good mood makes people see others and events in a positive light, and it's not surprising that a playful spirit is a tool of intelligent leaders. These authors refer to studies which show that the more positive the general mood of top management teams, the greater the cooperation between the members of each group and the better the results of the company's activity. Percentage-wise, the same authors refer to a ratio of: "for every 1% improvement in the working environment, there is a 2% increase in profits" (Idem, p.35). These same authors (Idem), give an example applied to the nursing professional group, concluding that in coronary intensive care units, where the general mood of the nurses was characterized as *depressed*, the mortality rate of patients was higher than in other similar units.

When we talk about the position of leader, we necessarily have to talk about self-assessment, so that the leader also has a realistic view of their performance. Goleman, Boyat/is and McKee (2002) assume that the higher up the hierarchical ladder a leader goes, the more difficult their self-assessment becomes, while at the same time there is a huge lack of access to other people's opinions and *feedback*. If this happens, the leader or head nurse will have more obstacles to evaluate the leader-member relationship and, consequently, modify the type of relationship and consideration for the emotions of subordinates (Dias, 2005). According to Goleman, Boyatzis and McKee (2002), it is not easy for a manager to know what others think, especially when it comes to the way in which management itself is carried out. The same authors point out that the paradox lies in the fact that the higher the leader's position in the organization, the more they need the reactions of others, but people suppress information when it is negative, for fear of reprisals from their bosses. The problem of lack of *feedback* is even greater when the leaders are female or belong to ethnic minorities, and it is noted that the leaders themselves do not ask their employees for their opinions, believing that even if they did get them, they would be useless because they would not be able to change (Goleman, Boyatzis and McKee, 2002). Self-awareness and self-assessment thus become extremely important skills in leaders, depending crucially on obtaining frank and open information about their leadership qualities.

Learning to be a resonant leader

EI competencies and resonant styles are not innate skills, they are acquired abilities that can be taught and learned throughout life and can be retained in the long term (Goleman, 2003). It is true that there is a genetic element to EI, but learning also plays a role, and there are examples of leaders who have made significant changes to the way they lead and sometimes even changed their personal lifestyles (Goleman, Boyatzis and McKee, 2002).

According to Goleman, Boyatzis and McKee (2002), self-directed learning is based on five discoveries, with the aim of using each of these discoveries as a tool to make the changes that are necessary for a person to become emotionally intelligent, in the eighteen leadership competencies, divided into the four major domains mentioned above. To summarize, people who succeed in the process of self-transformation, triggering or continuing the effective development of EI, with lasting effects, go through the following phases (Goleman, Boyatzis and McKee, 2002):

- The first discovery: the ideal me - how do I want to be? This is the beginning of change and it requires self-awareness;
- The second discovery: the real me - what am I like? What are my strengths and shortcomings?
- The third discovery: the learning program - reinforcing strengths and reducing shortcomings;
- The fourth discovery: reprogramming the brain. Experiment with new behaviors, thoughts and feelings until you master them completely;
- The fifth breakthrough: developing trusting relationships that support change and make it possible (the power of interpersonal relationships).

Thus, existing research shows that great leaders make themselves, that is, throughout their lives and professional careers, they acquire the skills that make them more efficient. In the professional practice of nursing, and in the organizations where nurses work, this is no exception. At operational management level, the leadership styles of head nurses influence the motivation for the work carried out by nurses, leading them to greater balance and job satisfaction (Dias, 2005). This leads us to believe that a leader can be a head nurse but, conversely, a head nurse may not be a leader.

Chapter 7

7 - IN NURSING EDUCATION

In the last decade, there has been a growing interest in developing school programs focused on EI skills (Mayer and Cobb, in press, Salovey and Sluyter, 1997, cited by Salovey, Mayer and Caruso, 2002). The typical characteristics of EI, particularly empathy, represent the basic structure of nursing care, both clinically and theoretically. However, their acquisition during basic training is increasingly compromised (Cadman and Brewer, 2001). According to these authors, these skills are best developed if there is a close teacher-student relationship, something that is increasingly difficult to achieve due to the growing number of students, the pressures exerted on teachers combined with clinical commitments and the need to research and publish work (Thomson 1999, cited by Cadman and Brewer, 2001). The reality described refers to the English context, but we can certainly find some parallels in our country. On the other hand, the development of these affective skills in the context of higher education could prove problematic, since market forces shape and limit both professional practice and the educational provisions of nursing. As a result, quality nursing practice is increasingly recognized only in terms of *mechanized* skills and the profitability of resources of various kinds (Cadman and Brewer, 2001).

With the changes in the health system, at all levels, the health technician (nurse) is faced with difficulties in responding to a wide variety of situations and problems, which are impossible to systematize in their entirety during basic training (Espiney et al., 2004).

As defined by the Order of Nurses (2003, p.5), in relation to the field of nursing intervention, the object of nursing study is "not the disease itself, but the human response to health problems and life processes as well as the transitions faced by individuals, families and groups throughout the life cycle". In other words, "nurses are expected to contribute towards increasing people's repertoire of internal resources to deal with challenges that require adaptation and self-control" (Espiney et al., 2004, p.7). Given these guidelines for nursing care providers, other questions arise:

> *Do nurses have the necessary skills to adapt to the multiple and complex situations arising from care processes?*

> *If they don't have these skills, how can nurses fulfill their social mission?*

Issues such as these underpin our recognition of the importance of developing EI skills in professional nursing practice. The idea is also reinforced by the working group on the implementation of the Bologna Process in nursing education, coordinated by Luísa d'Espiney, stating that:

> "Our history reveals the concern to invest in a generalist-based education that promotes the cultural, personal, social and ethical development of students, providing them with the scientific foundations to exercise a multifaceted activity that takes place in different social contexts, along with a strong investment in the development of the nursing discipline." (Espiney et al., 2004, p.8)

In this sense, Cadman and Brewer (2001) point out that selection processes are needed to determine the levels of EI in potential candidates, as these processes would offer reliable predictors of success both in nursing practice and in academic studies. Research indicates that EI cannot be developed quickly enough through interpersonal skills training. Studies indicate that characteristics such as the ability to motivate others, communicate convincingly and resolve conflicts are not found in the *helping professions* (Cadman and Brewer, 2001). The ability to empathize is seen as a fundamental aspect of EI, but Wheeler and Barret (1994, cited by Cadman and Brewer, 2001) recorded low levels of empathy in nursing teachers and other studies indicate that levels remain low in many areas of nursing practice (MacKay et al., 1990, Reynolds, 1998, cited by Cadman and Brewer, 2001). This raises the question of whether there are in fact training models capable of developing this capacity in students. It would therefore be rational to recruit students who already possess these skills or who at least demonstrate the potential to develop them, given that, in decision-making and intervention processes, feelings count as much, or perhaps even more, than thought (Cadman and Brewer, 2001). Based on this principle, the importance of EI as a criterion for selecting students and, consequently, for improving the quality of care provided, should be recognized and worked on. Proof of this is the fact that the inclusion of EI skills is increasingly being incorporated into the training of doctors (Kramer, Ber and Moores, 1989, cited by Salovey, Mayer and Caruso, 2002).

7.1 - CONTRIBUTIONS TO TRAINING

To enable a nursing student to develop their professional skills (making decisions, being aware, using ethics, taking responsibility and being autonomous), not only technical and cognitive skills are needed, but also emotional skills. All these skills are always implicit in the care process and the therapeutic relationship. They enable nurses to perform well professionally, to adapt better to the changes and particularities of the environment/team in which they work and also to provide more appropriate responses to the situations caused by the patients' clinical condition.

Knowing today that EI can be taught and learned throughout life (Goleman, 2003), it is up to nursing educators to incorporate the skills associated with EI into the expected competencies of the curriculum. It is also suggested that effective ways should be found or created to measure the extent to which these skills are acquired at the end of the nursing course, as is the case with cognitive and technical skills. Better work needs to be done on integrating emotional competencies throughout the nursing learning curriculum, rather than relying solely on transitional experiences at the end of training programs, such as clinical placements for integration into professional life.

At the level of initial and postgraduate training, pedagogical strategies should be used to promote the acquisition of relational and emotional skills in nursing professionals. Professional enrichment with this type of *tool* is essential if nursing students are to be able to overcome the difficulties inherent in their work.

Nursing schools must become the main protagonists of training concepts where *emotional literacy* is exposed and, before that, felt. As Branco (2004b) reports, it will be essential for this process to focus on the relational and emotional development of the practitioner (outlining the profiles of the practitioner/learner we want to achieve), and not just their technical-scientific skills (which are also very important). This formula could be the one that not only develops trainees in these skills, on a personal and professional level, but also the one that presents a truly pedagogical trainer.

Going a step further, we believe it is a priority to adopt a nursing entrance exam that also includes an assessment of EI skills, or the student's ability to learn how to develop the emotional competencies needed to practice the profession. Along these lines, the reflection group on the *Bologna declaration and the nursing trainee* proposed in its report that, in addition to the 12th year of schooling and the specific tests, a prerequisite for selection should be required in the area of "interpersonal communication" (Santos, Duarte and Subtil, 2004, p.24). By promoting EI skills through emotional education, it is possible not only to improve personal and/or group image, but also to optimize professional performance.

7.1.1 - The emotional education of nurses

Success in personal, professional and organizational life is too complex to depend solely on the emotional factor. However, it is now known that an emotionally competent person has greater potential to overcome problems and manage their life in a safer and more productive way (Goleman, 2003). The author, assuming that emotional intelligence (EI) skills are innate and crucial for optimizing professional performance, disseminates the news that, without the slightest doubt, emotional competence can be learned and improved throughout life.

Learning these skills, in other words, learning to be emotionally competent, is what the author calls *emotional literacy* (Goleman, 2003). Another researcher states that:

"Emotional literacy is just as important for learning and for technical-scientific training as any other subject, so emotions should be one of the subjects, in their own right, in the curriculum of schools and in the teaching philosophy of teachers." (Branco, 2004b, p.75)

In order to be happy, we don't need to wait for other people to make us feel good, because within each of us lies a world of possibilities that we may not know about and that we can take advantage of to achieve what we want (Galindo, 2003).

Emotional literacy can be developed in the context of academic training (undergraduate and postgraduate), as well as in work contexts. To do this, its promoters (teachers and nurses) need to adopt strategies and possess certain characteristics, which are discussed in this chapter.

With regard to emotional education, we are referring to two contexts that are both close and simultaneously distinct: the workplace and academic training, as well as a model for training trainers in EI.

7.1.1.1 - Academically

Ulla et al (cited by Colell Brunet et al., 2004) say that facing particularly delicate situations without specific training can lead to a reduction in the quality of care provided to patients and their families. The authors add that a more in-depth study of EI at the beginning of nursing courses (undergraduate) could help to provide better preparation for coping with the stress and anxiety generated when caring for patients, particularly the terminally ill.

One of the challenges in the training of future nursing professionals is to "prepare individuals for a high capacity to adapt to new professional situations that will inexorably arise in the course of each individual's career." (Portugal. Ministério da Saúde, 2000, p.31). Along the same lines as these guidelines, Carvalhal (2003) states that the teacher, the nurse tutor and the nursing student should interact towards a common goal, enabling and facilitating students to acquire different nursing knowledge and skills, so that they become the competent nurses we want them to be. The training of future professionals must allow for the correct appropriation of the skills that are indispensable to the practice of the profession, "(...) alongside a process of personal development towards a level of psychosocial and moral maturity that allows for the use of the *self* as a *therapeutic instrument*" (Santos, Duarte and Subtil, 2004, p.19). These competencies (cognitive, instrumental and socio-relational) are required by the Order of Nurses and are in line with the competencies included in the *Framework of Competencies for the Generalist Nurses of* the International Council of Nurses (Idem).

According to Bellack (1999), referring to the American context, there is already a lot of evidence that nursing pedag*ogues* are doing a good job with regard to the contents and pedagogies of the nursing curriculum. The author points out that officially published reports suggest that, collectively, courses and clinical experiences are continually being revised and corrected in order to align programs with the ever-changing health field. But unfortunately, says the author, this is not enough in today's working world. As far as we are concerned, there is a gap in this important area. Many of the social and emotional skills that are essential for success and proper performance in today's complex and demanding working environment are lacking in the training of students. However, in order to learn how to learn, whatever the circumstances in an interpersonal and inter-relational teacher/student activity, there needs to be "a reciprocal, asymmetrical and dialectical relationship between these subjects" (Tavares, 1993, cited by Branco, 2004b, p.20).

Nursing schools should dedicate part of their curricula to training skills that integrate tools for dealing with the adversities of a profession that cares for and interacts with people.

According to Espiney et al. (2004, p.11), "(...) the provision of health care places nurses in problematic situations that are characterized by unpredictability, uncertainty, disorder, (...)". According to Bellack (1999), unconventional learning experiences that reflect the realities of the working environment are needed in order to build students' emotional competence. For example: exams that have teamwork as a prerequisite to produce answers to certain questions and that reward students who manage to do so; active participation in healthcare teams (when experimenting with a clinical innovation); or confronting students with some kind of change. Cognitive abilities and technical skills are essential, but they are not enough to perform in a profession as complex as nursing.

From a perspective of developing students' social and emotional competence, it would not be logical to teach this content as therapy, but rather in a natural way and integrated into the pedagogical action (Branco, 2004b). This set of skills are "felt to be essential for achieving a level of autonomy and freedom, of expression and action, in the sense of being able to construct the Project of Self" (Antonovsky, 1995, De Jours, 1995, cited by Branco, 2004b, p.76).

Augusto et al. (2004) suggest, in the conclusions of a study entitled: "*The nurse's body in care practice - What meanings? What relationship?*", that nursing courses should include subjects that enable future nurses to reflect on and value the body in interpersonal relationships in the context of providing care. It is essential to act in order to develop in everyone "a taste for caring for their own body and image, as a form of personal appreciation, which would have repercussions in the pleasant recognition of their presence by others" (Idem, p.35).

Goleman (2000) believes that the training of health professionals should include at least some of the basic *tools of* EI, namely self-awareness, empathy and listening. At this point, we could say that it is important to invest in the equal development of the two types of intelligence: cognitive/intellectual and emotional. Neither is more important than the other, but both are fundamental.

Candidates for higher education are selected on the basis of their academic performance and their ability to succeed in exams, which tends to reflect patterns of IQ and convergent thinking. However, Gross (1992, cited by Cadman and Brewer, 2001) has documented that divergent thinking is an essential prerequisite for exceptional intellectual performance. Divergent thinkers tend to create a wide variety of new ideas and therefore perform better at solving problems that require creative solutions. They also tend to be more intuitive and are more likely to put their social intelligence into practice. Given the complex and pluralistic nature of nursing, a balance is needed between logical convergent thinking and divergent thinking (Idem and Ibidem). Although it is possible to work on a student's deficits with regard to EI, the time available to do so is insufficient, which is why it is necessary to reflect on the process of admitting students to nursing courses. The existence of a specific entrance exam, in our opinion, could be a good way of selecting the students with the best profile

to become a nurse. In addition to cognitive tests, personal and social skills tests should be applied, i.e. IQ and EQ tests (Cadman and Brewer, 2001). This prerequisite would thus guarantee that future nurses have the necessary tools for excellent professional performance. At present, this solution is no more than a hypothesis, as its application would be controversial to say the least.

Several factors have contributed to additional pressure on teachers and students. The significant increase in the *numerus clausus* for the nursing course and the demand for qualified nurses are just two examples. Students are increasingly required to guide their study, which can be very stressful for many, as qualities such as confidence and motivation are needed on a large scale and it is these same attributes that easily crumble under the pressure of academic study. Mayer and Kilpatrick (1994, cited by Cadman and Brewer, 2001) suggest that emotionally intelligent people are more likely to overcome the stress inherent in nursing practice, as well as that caused by individual study. Therefore, we should make sure that the nursing students we recruit demonstrate a strong potential to achieve good results in theory and practice. The presence of EI could be a strong indication of future good results in both spheres.

7.1.1.2 - In the workplace

The Order of Nurses (2003, p.188) defines the competence of general care nurses as "a level of professional performance that demonstrates the effective application of knowledge and skills, including judgment". This competence implies the use of skills that go beyond knowledge and techniques, falling into areas such as: professional, ethical and legal practice; the provision and management of care and professional development.

According to Bento (1997), the provision of health care is a complex reality, so the training of nurses should not only involve technical knowledge, but it is also essential that it promotes the development of the professional's personality, so that they can successfully adapt to all the demands that their professional performance requires. Thus, there are already trends that point to a commitment to emotional training and education. Proof of this are the studies in the context of leadership (Goleman, Boyatzis and McKee, 2002) which demonstrate the benefits of an emotionally intelligent leader.

Speaking of health professionals - *people who deal with people* - we think that the relevance of this topic is not just restricted to team managers or heads of human resources departments, but to all professionals at various levels of the hierarchy. But if the first situation arises, it's already a good starting point. According to Goleman, Boyatzis and McKee (2002), the development of emotional competencies, applied to increasing professional potential, helps to resolve problems and conflicts in the company, generate original ideas and create resonant orientations, leading to positive dialogues for optimizing performance. Organizations that invest in measures to develop emotional competencies will obtain greater satisfaction, personal appreciation and a consequent increase in the productivity of their employees (Idem). Augusto et al. (2004, p.35) also propose the creation of body expression classes and "a space for relaxation and physical and psychological care for professionals".

According to Bellack (1999), these skills require more than socializing newly graduated nurses or guiding them to become respectable members of a multi-professional team. EI is not about the profession itself and has to do with the world and the responsibilities behind the job. It is linked to a lifelong personal commitment to continuing education.

There are already several courses and trainings aimed at promoting the development of emotional skills. Their programs often include topics related to managing relationships and controlling emotions in the workplace. The limitation of these training courses is that they only reach the people who seek them out. It would be good if this type of training were promoted by the employers themselves and seen as a useful investment and a fundamental tool for improving the quality of the services provided. However, it seems obvious to us that emotional education and training programs should be adapted to both the group and the needs identified by managers and employees.

Goleman founded the Consortium for Research on Emotional Intelligence in Organizations. It is an association of researchers and professionals from management and administration faculties, the American Federal Government, consulting firms and other companies, which investigates scientific discoveries about changes in behavior, and analyzes training programs with a view to creating fundamental guidelines for the best procedures in teaching and training in *Emotional Competence* (Goleman, 2000). In Portugal too, it seems to us that it is imperative to give value to the development of emotional competences, both at the level of nursing undergraduates and at the level of continuing or post-graduate training, providing nurses with yet another tool to enable them to respond effectively to the challenges of the profession.

7.1.1.3 - The emotional trainer: an example

According to Bellack (1999), teachers, tutors and nurses who guide students on internships are educators responsible for training nurses. As such, they should be the ones to demonstrate that they have the necessary personal and social skills, and only then expect them from the students. This author leaves us with some topics that nursing teachers should look at and be prepared to improve on if they can't respond positively:

- Do I recognize and manage my emotions effectively?
- Do I know my strengths and limits?
- Can I be trusted?
- Do I take responsibility for my own performance?
- Am I comfortable with new ideas or suggestions? Am I open to new possibilities and willing to take on new opportunities? Am I flexible and willing to change?
- Am I optimistic? Am I persistent despite barriers or failures?
- Do I show interest and concern for others? Am I a good listener?
- I made a commitment to the development of my students, my nursing colleagues and myself?
- Am I willing to serve my patients, their families, students and employers?
- Do I value everyone's differences and the rich diversity of the people I work with?

- Am I an efficient team member? Do I contribute to common goals? Do I create synergies with other team members?

In Buenos Aires, there are already training courses in EI, such as the Curso de *Instructorado en Inteligencia Emocional - Un Aprendizaje Para Toda la Vida* (Cortese, 2005). This course lasts one year and has two levels: the first (six months) corresponds to *Mentoring* - Mentor, and the second level (six months) provides the degree of *Instructorado* - Instructor (Idem). According to its promoters, the course has various fields of application, including business organizations and educational and health institutions. The training methodologies are diverse, including: group dynamics, exercises and practical work (individual and group), the application of tests, visualization and analysis of literature, films, among others. In promoting the course, the coordinator lists some of the basic characteristics for becoming an *Emotional Mentor* or *Instructor*. With regard to the profile that *Mentors* (1st level) should have, Cortese (2005) states that:

- You must be a person who wants to have a positive influence on others;
- Someone who shares their knowledge and experience with others;
- Their presence provides support, advice, friendship, strength and constructive examples that lead to personal and group triumph;
- Your presence can mean the difference between success and failure;
- She is a person with great knowledge and wisdom, who shares experiences with younger people, also called protégés, helping them to develop their own abilities - on a personal and professional level;
- It offers a wide view;
- He's willing to listen;
- He has leadership experience;
- Shows a genuine interest in others;
- Show patience and affection;
- You have faith in other people's abilities;
- He is sensitive to the needs and circumstances of others;
- He is willing to motivate young people to grow and learn;
- He has a sense of humor;

- Make strong personal commitments to the relationship;
- They have the ability to accept different points of view.

At the level of the *Emotional Instructor* (2nd), and still according to the same author (Cortese, 2005), there are some requirements that must be met:

- Who wants to: it is vital that the instructor wants to share knowledge and experience with others and enjoys doing so;
- Let them know: no one can teach what they don't know;
- That you know how: just mastering a subject doesn't guarantee that you can communicate it in a pedagogical way. A person can be a master of a particular subject, but a terrible lecturer. *Knowing how will* enable the trainer to be competent in the use and variation of effective techniques for a given objective;
- Know how adults learn: mastering audiovisual techniques and resources helps the trainer to reduce barriers and make the participants' learning a success;
- Who knows how to communicate: it is difficult for people to retain and understand abstract concepts. Images, on the other hand, are content that is better retained and easily assigned meaning.

In conclusion, the *Instructor* has the responsibility to use all the means at his disposal, as well as having the ability to lead, stimulate and help the group to achieve its objectives, favoring learning and the development of EI skills (Cortese, 2005).

This two-year course model, developed by Abel Cortese's team, could be a guideline for the creation of training courses and programs for nurses, both in the workplace and at the academic level. In terms of basic training for nurses, it would be important for schools to include lectures on managing and educating emotions in their programs. In healthcare organizations too, it's up to managers (at both top and middle levels) to develop strategies for emotional education, so that their staff can develop clinical practices that are effective in dealing with the complex situations they face.

It makes more and more sense to publicize the benefits of personal skills which, according to Goleman, Boyatzis and McKee (2002), we can all learn at any stage of life, using them to improve relationships and the productivity of individuals in the most varied environments and organizational contexts. In the future, psychological intervention in professional contexts could be a reality, diagnosing, promoting and developing the emotional competencies of people in the organization.

At the end of this sub-chapter, we are left with a question: *How can we continue to innovate teaching-learning strategies so that our students become more emotionally, cognitively and technically competent nurses?*

The answer to this question would be a research project in itself. However, we hope that by reading this book you will be able to glimpse some possibilities for development and intervention.

Chapter 8

8 - THE EMOTIONALLY COMPETENT NURSE

Emotional intelligence (EI) has implications not only for personal life, but also for the practice of a profession such as nursing. Not only in the performance of its social function, but also in everything that surrounds it, such as: the training of professionals, the way they are managed (at all levels), as well as in the organizations where they work. The following chapter will look at the contributions and implications of EI for nursing professionals. Authors will be mentioned, mainly foreign ones, who have already addressed the issue.

According to the Order of Nurses (2003, cited by Espiney et al., 2004, p.9), the professional practice of nursing "focuses on the interpersonal relationship between a nurse and a person, or between a nurse and a group of people (family or community) (...). The therapeutic relationship (...) is characterized by the partnership established with the client, with respect for their abilities (...) and (...) is part of a context of multi-professional action".

Since nursing is considered a "meaningful, therapeutic and interpersonal" process (Peplau, 1952, p.16, cited by Cadman and Brewer, 2001), the recognition that nursing professionals must be competent in dealing with their own and others' emotions is indisputable. The emotional state of the patient/client is often altered during illness, particularly in serious illnesses, as mental sanity is partly based on the illusion of invulnerability (Goleman, 2003). According to Cadman and Brewer (2001), this illusion can fade quickly, making the person feel vulnerable and anxious. Nursing professionals must therefore be able to respond with empathy, kindness and genuine concern.

Nurses in Portugal, as in other countries in the Western world, are facing increasing challenges related to "the complexity of health and illness situations that require an interdisciplinary approach, which goes beyond the health area and requires real teamwork (...), to overcome internal and external obstacles to the organization where they work" (Santos, Duarte and Subtil, 2004, p.4). Among the various challenges that these authors pose to the nursing profession, and the health professions in general, we cite (Idem and Ibidem):

- "The challenge of the CARE paradigm, from a health perspective, as a necessity for Humanity, (...) requiring true multidisciplinary teamwork;
- New health problems related to lifestyles, ageing, chronic diseases, AIDS/HIV, drug addiction and social exclusion, among others;
- Change in the care landscape (...) by transferring hospital care to community services and reorganizing primary health care. (...);
- The increasing complexity of the professional situations to be managed and the evolution of work organization (...) implies the emergence of <collective competence> resulting from the quality of cooperation between individual competences;
- (...) related to citizens' rights and duties, diversity, differentiation and multiculturalism;

■ (...) and the need for new strategies for a new positioning of the school and the profession (...), in which <lifelong learning> is the dominant motto".

Martins et al. (2003) add that nursing today is going through times of change, with technological advances, new diseases and different demands from health organizations and different care needs from users. These authors felt the need to reflect on how necessary it is to exercise these emotional intelligence (EI) skills. All these skills are considered essential for efficient nursing practice (MacCormack, 1993, Taylor, 1994, cited by Cadman and Brewer, 2001). It seems obvious to assume that emotionally competent individuals make a positive contribution to their workplace, voicing concerns such as quality, improved patient care outcomes and staff recruitment and management (Cadman and Brewer, 2001).

At this point, we wonder what a nurse's *life* is like, and what the employer/organization gains when, in the course of their professional practice, a professional: faces career progression obstacles; is in the type of service for which they don't feel motivated; has no incentive to continue their training; doesn't feel a true and genuine team spirit; behaves like a hostile professional because they don't feel their work is recognized; is overworked and not rewarded; doesn't achieve success in the care they provide, among others. On the other hand, Espiney et al. (2004, p.11) state that, in order to perform well professionally, nurses are expected to be able to integrate the specific skills of the profession, together with another group of "transversal skills which include flexibility, creativity, autonomy, a sense of responsibility, teamwork, adaptation to change, the ability to reflect critically, to make decisions and the ability to act competently and autonomously within a multidisciplinary team". It is between what is expected and the reality perceived in practice that emotional - interpersonal and social competences come into play. A nurse who integrates all these skills is undoubtedly not only an excellent professional, but also an emotionally competent nurse. In this context, an initial question arises:

How important is emotional intelligence in professional nursing practice?

According to Salovey, Mayer and Caruso (2002), EI can be an important predictor of success in personal relationships, in the family and in the workplace. In a wide variety of contexts, the validity of EI is increasingly being developed due to the recognition of its usefulness. The role of EI in nurses' professional performance is emphasized by authors such as Goleman (2000, 2003), Jesus (2004), Bellack (1999), Cadman and Brewer (2001), Vitello-Cicciu (2003) and Colell Brunet et al. (2004). The main conceptual reference for this work, Goleman (2003, p.54), states that: "At best, IQ contributes about 20 percent to the factors that determine success in life, which leaves 80 percent for other forces." On the other hand, and emphasizing the importance of EI, Jesus (2004), in one of his studies, suggests that nurses with higher levels of EI may have better professional performance. The concepts of professional nursing practice encompass not only technical issues but also a fusion of clinical skills, care and a relationship with users, clients and other professionals.

(Halldorsdottir 1996, cited by Cadman and Brewer, 2001).

Referring back to the importance of recognizing EI skills in nurses' professional performance, we reinforce the importance of managers' involvement in facilitating and developing these skills, by setting up, for example, discussion and training groups on the behaviors and attitudes that teams show when faced with a given professional situation. In service meetings or training sessions, understanding and sharing the team's feelings could be a focus for enrichment, in order to reduce professional stress, hostility and professional isolation, among other benefits.

If working institutions or nursing schools don't provide the conditions for developing and learning these skills, it's up to each individual to feel the need to develop and train themselves. The gains that can be made will not only be for the individual, but also for the patient, the group and the whole organization.

CONCLUSION

The bibliographical review provides an overview of the relevance of Emotional Intelligence in the nursing profession. This framework was based on concepts inherent to EI, allowing us to refer to the main theoretical models, namely Goleman's - on which much of the research produced is based. We also had the opportunity to learn about other studies (particularly American and Spanish) on the influence of EI on nurses in various areas of its application, which enriched the discussion of the results obtained from the sample of nurses we studied. With regard to the results obtained in the study we presented, carried out in Portugal, we can see that some of these results are in line with those obtained in other studies, although the opposite was also true. Due to the frequency with which the results appear, the importance of age in influencing EI factors and abilities stands out. This is validated by Goleman himself (2000, 2003), who attaches great importance to *maturity in the* development of emotional competence. In this sample, it can be said that maturity, measured by advancing age and longer life experiences (personal and professional), determines the development of EI skills (particularly empathy and managing relationships in groups), helping nurses to overcome the difficulties arising from their work.

Overall, the sample surveyed perceived themselves as emotionally intelligent *infrequently*, with a strong tendency towards the *norm*. However, as this is not a homogeneous concept (as it includes five abilities), the nurses studied should improve these EI abilities, as their averages are below what we believe is desirable.

Although EI is a fragmented construct and is operationalized in five capacities, in this study they were correlated and with different frequencies, according to the theoretical model we adopted. The results obtained with our sample show that the five capabilities of EI, made up of the specific grouping of factors, are not homogeneous and equal to the theoretical construct. However, they correlate positively and significantly with each other and with Emotional Intelligence, but not in the same way as Goleman's (2000, 2003) theoretical model advocates.

The sample showed two types of skills: intrapersonal - which determine how nurses manage themselves, and interpersonal - which determine how nurses deal with relationships. The former are generally carried out with more negative attitudes and behaviors, according to the sample. The latter (interpersonal skills) are produced through positive behaviors and attitudes. There are also areas in which the sample of nurses does not perceive themselves as frequently as might be expected. For these reasons, and from our point of view, a better understanding of this phenomenon requires further research in the professional nursing group.

We found variables that seem to influence the factors, abilities and overall Emotional Intelligence of nurses. However, the size of the sample does not allow us to generalize the results on a national scale, only to the size of the organization where the study took place. However, taking into account the similarity of the socio-professional characteristics of this sample with the population of nurses nationwide, we can infer the possibility of some degree of external validity of the results. If this is true, it could be said that the results of this sample are useful for understanding the emotional competencies of nurses in Portugal, and could also be used to define training and management strategies for nurses at a national level.

We would like to point out that this is the emotional profile of the nurses studied, and we do not want to claim that it is generalizable to the universe of Portuguese nurses. We admit that when studying another sample of nurses, other differences may be found. The sample's responses reveal a **new and original configuration of emotional competence**, which concerns the emergence of a contextual profile, only possible in this sample of nurses and in their specific work contexts, which gives it unique and unrepeatable characteristics.

These results could show different paths for other research in the area of nurses' professional, personal and social competences, and constitute a small contribution to an area as vast and complex as human resource management - in the organizational contexts of work and initial and continuing training. In this sense, it must always be assumed that there are behavioral factors that lead to emotional competence, and that these are very relevant when it comes to nurses' training and management contexts.

We consider it increasingly important to include emotional skills in the nurse's profile, alongside technical and cognitive skills. The results, which differ somewhat from Goleman's theoretical proposal, are nevertheless a way of getting to know a reality. This is perhaps yet another challenge for nurse training, particularly in terms of defining competency profiles and their impact on professional performance.

With this work, we hope to have contributed to the knowledge of the variables related to emotional intelligence and to have raised awareness of the need not to neglect the importance of this type of intelligence in the success of the working lives of nurses, their own trainers, teams, managers and organizations and, consequently, the quality of care provided to users.

In carrying out this project, there were some difficulties, both theoretical and practical, which we feel should be mentioned.

FINAL REFLECTION

We believe that the research already carried out in this area, and what is explored in this document, has reciprocity and is pertinent from the top of management, through the operational level, to the care practices developed by nursing professionals. It could be the beginning, and a contribution, to the definition of an emotional intelligence assessment tool to help in the selection and recruitment of nursing professionals, giving them job opportunities suited to their profiles. The validation of the data collection instrument in this population also serves to increase the fidelity of this scale and make it possible to use it with other people/professionals.

We hope that this work can be an incentive to explore the importance of EI in *care professionals*. In this regard, management bodies have a key role to play in stimulating and developing these skills in these professionals, adopting emotional education and training strategies. By identifying these profiles, we believe that this information can be used to train nurses in skills that are still underdeveloped, but which are important given the specific nature of the services in which they work. In our opinion, the data collected is particularly important, not only for a better understanding of what emotionally involves these professionals, but also because it provides us with fundamental information for future emotional support and education projects in work contexts.

We believe that the analysis of behavior and emotions is a key factor in more effective human resources management. This obviously applies not only to nurses, but also to all other health professionals. Knowledge of emotional competencies in professionals complements and improves management skills, as it provides a more comprehensive view of everything that encompasses organizational contexts, including *people*.

Becoming aware of our EI abilities is a step towards living a better quality of life - professionally and personally. Using these abilities properly is a way of living better with others and giving meaning to life.

In this book, an attempt has been made to explain how EI skills are suited to the professional nursing context, pointing out that managers and organizations themselves, including Nursing Schools, can become enablers of the development of EI skills, with major positive effects on the efficiency and performance of nursing professionals. We also hope to have shown that EI is an excellent contribution to resonant leadership - the main task of leaders - considering primal leadership as a crucial dimension, which determines a large part of the success or failure of the leader's efforts.

It's important for managers of healthcare organizations to take a forward-looking view in developing strategies to help their employees, specifically nurses, feel better and be more competent in carrying out their duties. For us, being more competent means that each professional has the ability to deal with themselves and the people they relate to (personally or professionally).

Furthermore, as Bellack (cited by Colell Brunet et al, 2004) points out, the need to develop EI skills has made it possible to incorporate this subject into the syllabuses of some American nursing schools. We have no doubt that developing these skills can be one of the best ways of coping with the stress generated by working with the disease and the various problems that caring for users can bring.

The results found in this study suggest that professionals with certain *emotional intelligence profiles perform* better when they work in an area or type of service for which they have the greatest aptitude. In order to put this idea into practice, it is necessary that, in the future, nurses are allocated to health units according to their profile, not only technical but also emotional. This proposed approach can be implemented *a priori*, in the recruitment and selection of nurses, or *a posteriori*, through the redeployment of staff (negotiated between the manager and the employee) or emotional training, with regard to the development of emotional skills in which nurses show deficiencies.

By identifying the emotional profiles of nurses, it will be possible to train nurses in the EI skills that they have underdeveloped (adapting them to the particularities of their work context), and to select, redeploy and recruit nursing professionals in order to give them work opportunities suited to their profiles.

With the results of this study, we hope to help better understand the scope of emotional intelligence in promoting a work environment conducive to better professional *performance, as* well as contributing to the development of a philosophy centered on valuing the *human factor* within healthcare organizations. We believe that people with higher EI are more likely to succeed in life and find it easier to solve problems, which to others may seem like a very complicated task.

EI is a fundamental factor for the harmony of the human being as a person, educator and professional. As such, it is extremely important to extend studies in this area to a larger scale, both for nurses and other health professionals.

PROPOSALS FOR FUTURE STUDIES

The development of emotional intelligence is still at an early stage. According to Salovey, Mayer and Caruso (2002), what this area needs, as well as the general public, is researchers who treat their studies with the utmost empirical attention, so that the results are reliable and useful for families, schools, workplaces and even social relationships.

In an attempt to increase recognition of the importance of EI in nurses' work contexts, it would be interesting to continue research in this area. In particular, for the professional field of nursing, it would be very important to extend research to a national scale. If this extension is not possible, it would perhaps be pertinent for other studies to be carried out on populations of nurses in other regions of the country, in order to be able to triangulate and obtain more consistent data on the emotional competence of these professionals.

Believing in the above-mentioned statements, we pose some questions that we would like to see answered in the future. They are:

Will the best nursing students subsequently become the best professionals?

What qualities do employers and those responsible for recruiting nurses value in nursing professionals?

What qualities do citizens/users value in nursing professionals?

What influence do nurses' emotional competencies have on satisfaction with nursing care?

What is the motivation of nurses related to their perception of the leadership styles of middle managers?

While recent research in Portugal suggests that empathy has no explanatory value for the EI of the nurses studied, is the same true for other groups of nurses?

Organizations that see their employees as active agents in achieving their mission are generally more productive and more likely to succeed. This means that managers (operational, middle and/or top) need to recognize the emotional dimension in people in order to optimize their professional performance.

It is essential to understand professionals and *use* their constructive attitudes so that they can actively contribute to the collective's objectives and image. Managers need to understand the strategic usefulness of these concepts and invest in developing skills in the emotional sphere too.

When it comes to people management, it's important to know how your employees feel and live their professional practices. With this knowledge, you can define methodologies to improve the performance and, progressively, the *outputs of* your organization. These strategies are not expensive and certainly become measures that lead to profitability in production and improve the quality of the services provided, both individually and globally.

At the end of this work, we are aware that the methodological steps have been treated with the utmost rigor and scientific truth. We hope that we have contributed to increasing knowledge in the area of people management, particularly among nursing professionals. We also hope to have added clues to the development of management and training strategies for nurses, as health technicians, in order to facilitate an organizational climate that is more conducive to best professional practices.

We believe that more emotionally competent nurses will not only benefit themselves and their organizations, but above all the citizens, who will receive personalized, higher quality nursing care.

BIBLIOGRAPHY

ALBARELLO, L. [et al.] - *Practices and methods of research in social sciences.* Lisbon: Gradiva, 1997.

ALMEIDA, Leandro S.; FREIRE, Teresa - *Metodologia da Investigando em Psicología e Educando.* 2ª ed. rev. aument. Braga: Psiquilíbrios, 2000.

ALMEIDA, M. H. F. - Quality in health. *Ordem dos Enfermeiros.* N° 3, (2001), p. 39-40.

ALVAREZ GONZÁLEZ, M. [et al.] - *Design and evaluation of emotional education programs.* Barcelona: Cisspraxis, SA, 2001.

ANTUNES, Celso - *El desarrolo de la personalidad y la inteligencia emocional: Diálogos que ayudan a crecer.* Barcelona: Gedisa Editorial, 2000.

ASIAN, M. C. - Quantitative research. In DIEGO, M. C. *Investigación: su lugar en la prática de enfermaria.* Navarra: University School of Nursing. Clínica Universitaria de Navarra, 1995.

AUGUSTO [et al.] - The nurse's body and the practice of care. What meanings? What relationship? In *Percursos de investigando.* Coimbra: Formasau - Formagao e Saúde, 2004. p. 23-36.

BARDIN, Laurence - *Content analysis.* Lisbon: Edigoes 70, 1995.

BARRETT, L. F [et al.] - Are Women the More Emotional Sex? Evidence From Emotional Experience in Social Context. *Cognition and Emotion*, Vol. 12, n° 4 (1998), p. 555 - 578.

BELL, Judith - *How to carry out a research project.* Lisbon: Gradiva, 1997.

BELLACK, Janis P. - Emotional intelligence: A missing ingredient? *Journal of Nursing Education.* Vol. 38, n° 38 (Jan. 1999), p. 3-4.

BENTO, J. O. - The pedagogical act and teacher training. *Educagao.* No. 3 (1991), p. 96-99.

BENTO, M. C. - *Nursing care and training - what identity?* Lisbon: Fim de Século, 1997.

BERNARDO, A. S. S.; GOMES, I. D.; ALMEIDA, M. P. P. - Analysis of practices: A strategy for constructing knowledge in the practice of nursing care. *Formar: Revista dos Formadores.* Lisbon. N° 46-50 (Mar. 2004), p. 42-52.

BOGDAN, R.; BIKLEN, S. - *Qualitative research in education: an introduction to method theory.* Porto: Porto Editora, 1994.

BORGES, Livia Oliveira [et al.] - Burnout Syndrome and Organizational Values: A Comparative Study in University Hospitals. *Psychology: Reflection and Criticism.* Vol. 15, n° 1 (2002), p. 189-200.

BOWLING, A. - *La Medida De La Salud: Revision de las escalas de medida de la calidad de vida.* Barcelona: Masson, 1994, p.117-119. Translation of the original in English Measuring health: A review of quality of life measurement scales. Buckingham: Open University Press.

BRADBERRY, T.; GREAVES, J. - *Emotional Intelligence Appraisal - There is more than IQ* (Technical Manual) [online]. [consulted. 11 Aug. 2003]. Available at WWW:<URL: http://www.talentsmart.com>.

BRANCO, Maria Augusta Veiga - *Self-Motivation*. Coimbra: Quarteto, 2004a.

BRANCO, Maria Augusta Veiga - *Teacher emotional competence: From theoretical constructs to perceived reality*. Vila Real: [s.n.], 1999. Dissertation for the Master's Degree in Health Promotion/Education presented to the University of Trás-os-Montes and Alto Douro.

BRANCO, Maria Augusta Veiga - *Competencia Emocional em Professores: Um Estudo em Discursos do Campo Educativo*. Porto: [s.n.], 2005. Thesis for the degree of Doctor of Psychology and Educational Sciences presented to the University of Porto.

BRANCO, Maria Augusta Veiga - *Competencia Emocional: Um estudo com professores*. Coimbra: Quarteto, 2004b.

BRYMAN, A.; CRAMER, D. - *Data analysis in the social sciences: Introduction to techniques using SPSS*. Oeiras: Celta Editora, 1992.

BUENO, José Maurício Haas; PRIMI, Ricardo - Emotional intelligence: a validity study on the ability to perceive emotions. In *Psicología: Reflexao e Crítica*. Vol.16, n° 2 (2003). Porto Alegre. [consulted on May 10, 2005]. Available at WWW:<URL:http://www.scielo.br/scielo.php?script=sci arttext&pid=S 0102-7972200 3000200008#nt>.

BUZAN, Tony - *The Power of Intelligence*. Lisbon: Oficina do Livro, 2003.

CADMAN, C.; BREWER, J. - Emotional intelligence: a vital prerequisite for recruitment in nursing. *Journal of Nursing Management*. No. 9 (Feb. 2001), p. 321-324.

CARVALHAL, R. - *Expectations of students of the Higher Nursing Course in relation to nurse teachers: contribution to the knowledge of the expectations of the students of the Higher Nursing Course of the Angra do Heroismo Higher Nursing School*. Angra do Heroísmo: [s.n.], 1995. Dissertation presented as part of the Pedagogy Applied to Nursing Teaching course at the Angra do Heroísmo Nursing School.

CARVALHAL, R. - *Partnerships in training - Role of clinical advisors: actors' perspectives*. Loures: Lusociencia, 2003.

CHERNISS, Cary - Social and Emotional Competence in the Workplace. In BAR-ON, Reuven; PARKER, James D. A. - *The Handbook of Emotional Intelligence: Theory, Development, Assessment, and Application at Home, School, and in the Workplace*. San Francisco: Jossey-Bass, 2000. p. 433-458.

CHERNISS, Cary. *Emotional Intelligence: What it is and Why it Matters*. [online]. [consulted. 11 Aug. 2003]. Available at WWW:<URL:http://www.eicons ortium.org/research/wath is emotional intelligence.htm>.

COLELL BRUNET, R. [et al.] - Implication of Emotional Intelligence in Palliative Care Professionals. In ENCUENTRO DE INVESTIGACIÓN

ENFERMERÍA, 8. *Libro* de *Ponencias*. Sevilla: Unidad de coordinación y desarrollo de la Investigación en Enfermería, 2004, p. 56-59.

CONANGLA MARÍN, Mm - Acompañar en un viaje emocional. *Revista Rol de Enfermería* . Vol. 27, n° 3 (2004), p.42-50.

CORTESE, Abel - *Instructorado en Inteligencia Emocional - Un Aprendizaje Para Toda la Vida.* [online]. [consult. 3 Jan. 2005]. Available at WWW:<URL:http://www.inteligencia-emotional.org/actividades/instructorado.htm>.

COSTA, Arminda. *Announcement of partnership for the development of health training* [online message] to Carlos Vilela. [consult. 20 Jan. 2005].

DAMÁSIO, António R. - *Descartes' Error - Emondo, Razdo e Cérebro Humano.* Lisbon: Círculo de Leitores, 1995.

DAMÁSIO, António R. - *O sentimento de si - O Corpo, a Emondo e a Neurobiologia da Consciência.* 9ª ed. Mem Martins: Publicares Europa-América Lda., 2000.

DANIEL, Liliana Felcher - *Interpersonal attitudes in nursing.* São Paulo: E.P.U. - Editora Pedagógica e Universitária, 1983.

DANIEL, Liliana Felcher - *Interpersonal attitudes in nursing.* São Paulo: E.P.U. - Editora Pedagógica e Universitária Lda., 1983.

DESHAIES, B. - *Metodologia da investigando em ciencias humanas.* Lisbon: Instituto Piaget, 1992.

DIAS, Carlos Melo - Leadership in Nursing. In *Revista Portuguesa de Enfermagem.* Amadora: IFE - Instituto de Formagão Enfermagem, Lda., 2005. p. 46-52.

DURÁN ESCRIBANO, Marta - The power of values: A question of professionalism. *Revista Rol de Enfermería.* Vol. 27, n° 3 (2004), p.31-40.

ECO, U. - *How to write a thesis in the humanities.* 7ª ed. Lisbon: Editorial Presenta, 1998.

ELLIOT, Thomas [et al.] - Design and validation of instruments to measure knowledge. *Journal of Cancer Education,* Vol. 16, n° 3 (2001), p.157.

ESPINEY, Luisa d' [et al.]. Implementation of the Bologna Process at national level: Groups by Area of Knowledge - Nursing: report. [s. l.: s. n.], Dec. 2004.

FERNANDES, C.; REGO, A. - *How emotional intelligence explains students' life satisfaction and physical ill-health.* [online]. [consult. 28 Sept. 2004] Available at WWW:<URL: *http://brs.leeds.ac.uk/~beiww/BEIA/ecer2004.htm*>.

FERNANDES, C.; REGO, A. - *Emotional intelligence and students' academic performance: An empirical study in university education.* [online]. [Consult. 28 Sept. 2004]. Available at WWW:<URL: http://webct2.ua.pt/ public/leies/daes ie.pdf>.

FERNANDES, C.; REGO, A. - *Emotional intelligence and students' academic performance* (poster). [online]. [consult. 28 Sept. 2004]. AvailableWWW:<URL: http://webct2.ua.pt/public/leies/daes IE poster. pdf>.

FERNÁNDEZ-BERROCAL, P. [et al.] - Cultura, inteligencia emocional percibida y ajuste emocional: un estudio preliminar. [online]. *Revista Electrónica de Motivación y Emoción*. Vol. 4, n° 8-9 (2001). [consulted. 2 Oct. 2004] Available at WWW:<URL: http://reme.uji.es/reme/numero8-9/indexsp.html>.

FERNÁNDEZ-BERROCAL, P.; EXTREMERA PACHECO, N. - La inteligencia emocional como una habilidad esencial en la escuela. *Revista Iberoamericana de Educación*. Vol. 29, n° 1-6 (2002).

FERREIRA, Pedro Lopes; MARQUES, Francisco Batel - *Psychometric Evaluation and Cultural and Linguistic Adaptation of Health Measurement Instruments: General Methodological Principles: Working Paper*. Coimbra: University of Coimbra, Faculty of Economics, Center for Health Studies and Research, 1998.

FODDY, W. - *How to ask: theory and practice of constructing questions in interviews and questionnaires*. Oeiras: Celta Editora, 1996.

FONSECA, A. M. - What training for the 21st century? Some avenues for reflection.... *Formar*. N° 15, (1995), p. 44 - 49.

FORNÉS, J. [et al.] - Psychological Hostility in Nursing. Factorial Analysis of the HPT Questionnaire. In ENCUENTRO DE INVESTIGACIÓN ENFERMERÍA, 8. *Libro de Ponencias*. Sevilla: Unidad de coordinación y desarrollo de la Investigación en Enfermería, 2004, p. 317-318.

FORTIN, Marie-Fabienne - *The research process: from conception to realization*. Loures: Lusociencia, 1999.

FORTIN, Marie-Fabienne - *The research process: from conception to realization*. 2ª ed. Loures: Lusociencia, 2000.

GALINDO, Antonio - *Inteligencia emocional para jóvenes: Programa práctico de entrenamiento emocional*. Madrid: Prentice Hall, 2003.

GANDUM, Alexandre; PEDRO, Fernanda - Living on the edge. *Única: magazine of the Expresso newspaper*. Lisbon, (25 Mar. 2005), p. 66-71.

GASQUET - *Satisfaction des patients et perfomance hospitalere* [online]. Masson. [consulted. Jan. 2000]. Available at WWW:<URL: http://www.atmedica.com/article>.

GHIGLIONE, Rodolphe; MATALON, Benjamín - *Inquiry: Theory and Practice*. 4ª ed. Oeiras: Celta Editora, 2001.

GOLEMAN, Daniel - *Foreword*. In BAR-ON, Reuven; PARKER, James D. A..*The Handbook of Emotional Intelligence: Theory, Development, Assessment, and Application at Home, School, and in the Workplace*. San Francisco: Jossey-Bass, 2000. p. VII-XV.

GOLEMAN, Daniel - *Inteligência Emocional* - 12th ed. Lisbon: Temas e Debates, 2003.

GOLEMAN, Daniel - *Working with Emotional Intelligence*. - 3rd ed. Lisbon: Temas e Debates, 2000.

GOLEMAN, Daniel; BOYTZIS, Richard; McKEE, Annie - *The New Leaders: Emotional Intelligence in Organizations*. Lisbon: Gradiva, 2002.

HEDLUND, Jennifer; STERNBERG, Robert J. - Too Many Intelligences?

Integrating Social, Emotional, and Practical Intelligence. In BAR-ON, Reuven and PARKER, James D. A. - *The Handbook of Emotional Intelligence: Theory, Development, Assessment, and Application at Home, School, and in the Workplace.* San Francisco: Jossey-Bass, 2000. p. 136-167.

HILL, Manuela Magalhaes; HILL, Andrew - *Research by questionnaire*. Lisbon: Edigoes Sílabo, 2002.

Emotional Intelligence at the Service of Companies and Teams. [online]. [consulted. 29 Apr. 2004]. Available at WWW:<URL: http://www.dashofer.pt/e-newsletters/pdf inteligencia.jsp.>.

Emotional INTELLIGENCE. [online]. [consulted 12 Apr. 2005]. Available at WWW:<URL: http://www.inteligencia-emociona⁻.org/>.

INTERNATIONAL TEST COMMISSION (ITC) - International *Guidelines for the Use of Tests* (Portuguese Version: Commission for the Portuguese Adaptation of the International Guidelines for the Use of Tests). [online]. [consult. 12 Aug. 2004]. Available   inWWW   :<URL: http://www.intestcom.org/Downloads/Portuguese %20guidelines%202003.pdf>.

JACQUES, S. M. C. - *Biostatistics: principles and applications*. Porto Alegre: Artmed, 2003.

JESUS, Élvio Henriques - *Patterns of cognitive ability and clinical decision-making in nursing*. Porto: [s.n.], 2004. Thesis for the degree of Doctor of Nursing Sciences at the University of Porto - Abel Salazar Institute of Biomedical Sciences.

KERLINGER, F. N. - *Metodologia da pesquisa em ciencias sociais*. Sao Paulo: E.P.U. - Editora Pedagógica e Universitária Lda., 1980.

LA INTELIGENCIA emocional en la salud [online]. [consult. 23 Dec. 2003]. Available at WWW:<URL: http://www.inteligencia- emocional.org/associacion/salud.htm>.

LAKATOS, E. M.; MARCONI, M. A. - *Metodologia do trabalho científico.* 2.ª ed. Sao Paulo: Editora Atlas, 1988.

LAKATOS, E. M.; MARCONI, M. A. - *Técnicas de pesquisa.* 2.ª ed. São Paulo: Editora Atlas, 1990.

LESSARD - HÉBERT, M.; GOYETTE, G.; BOUTIN, G. - *Investigaçäo Qualitativa: fundamentos e práticas*. Lisbon: Instituto Piaget, 1990.

LOPÉZ MILLANO, Elix; SULBARÁN, Mercedes - Diseño *de un programa de adiestramiento basado en Inteligencia Emocional: Para el personal del departamento de recursos humanos de la aduana principal de Marcaibo* [online]. [consult. 14 Feb. 2005]. Available at WWW:<URL: http://www.monografias.com/trabajos 16/adiestramiento/adiestramiento2.shtml>.

MAIA, Carlos Manuel Leitão - *Social representations of the functions performed by nurses in a district hospital*. Lisbon: [s.n.], 1995. Dissertation for the Master's Degree in Nursing Sciences at the Portuguese Catholic University - Faculty of Human Sciences.

MARROCO, João - *Statistical analysis using SPSS*. Lisbon: Edigoes Sílabo,

2003. p. 46.

MÄRTIN, Doris; BOECK, Karin - *EQ: What is Emotional Intelligence?* 2nd ed. Lisbon: Editora Pergaminho, Lda., 1999.

MARTINS, Fernando [et al.] - Emotional intelligence - a challenge for nursing. *Nursing.* Lisbon. N° 176 (Apr. 2003), p. 28-30.

MAYER, John D. - *Emotional Intelligence Information* [online]. [consulted. 12 Jan. 2005]. Available at WWW:<URL: http://www.unh.edu/emotional intelligence /index.html>.

MAYER, John; SALOVEY, Peter - *Emotional Development and Emotional Intelligence: Educational Implications.* New York: Basic Books, 1997.

MAYER, Jonh D. [et al.] - Measuring Emotional Intelligence With the MSCEIT V2.0. *Emotion.* Vol. 3, n° 1 (2003), p.97-105.

MESTRE NAVAS, P. [et al.] - Cuando los constructos psicológicos escapan del método científico: El caso de la inteligencia emocional y sus implicaciones en la validación *y* evaluación [online] *Revista Electrónica de Motivación y Emoción.* Vol. 3, n° 4 (2000). Available at WWW:<URL: http://reme.uji.es/reme /numero4/indexsp.html>.

MIRANDA, Roberto Lira - *Beyond Emotional Intelligence: Integral use of brain skills in learning, work and life.* [online]. [consulted. 11 Aug. 2003]. Available at WWW:<URL: http://www.editoras.com/campus/ 20184.htm>.

MOREIRA, José Manuel - *Accounts with Business Ethics.* Cascais: PRINCIPIA, Publicagoes Universitárias e Científicas, 1999.

NETO, Luís Miguel; MARUJO, Helena Águeda - *Optimism and Emotional Intelligence: A Guide for Educators and Leaders.* 2ª ed. Lisbon: Editorial Presenga, 2002.

OLÓRTEGUI YZU, Dante R. - *Administración de Recursos Humanos en Clínicas y Hospitales* [online]. [consult. 14 Feb. 2005]. Available at WWW:<URL: http://www.monografias.com/trabajos15/rrhh- hospitales/rrhh-hospitales. shtml>.

ORDER OF NURSES - Competencies of the general care nurse. Order of Nurses. N° 10 (2003), p. 49-56.

ORDEM DOS ENFERMEIROS - CONSELHO DE ENFERMAGEM - *From the Road Traveled and the Proposals (analysis of the first mandate - 1999/2003).* Lisbon: Order of Nurses, 2004.

ORDEM DOS ENFERMEIROS - CONSELHO DE ENFERMAGEM - *Padrões de Qualidade dos Cuidados de Enfermagem: Enquadramento conceptual - Enunciados descritivos*: relatório. [s.l.: s.n.], Dec. 2001.

ORDER OF NURSES - Nurses: a critical overview of the world. Ordem dos Enfermeiros. N° 10 (2003), p. 13.

PAGE, M. J. - *Elements of psychometrics.* Madrid: Endema, 1993.

PARKINSON, B. - What we Think about When we Think about Emotion? *Cognition and Emotion,* Vol.12, N° 4, (1998), p. 615 - 624.

PAÚL, C.; FONSECA, A.M. - *Psychosociology of Health*. Lisbon: Climepsi Editores, 2001.

PÉREZ GONZÁLES, Juan Carlos - *How can emotional intelligence be measured?* [online message] to Carlos Vilela. [consulted 30 Mar 2005].

PESTAÑA, Maria Helena; GAGEIRO, Joao Nunes - *Data Analysis for Social Sciences: the complementarity of SPSS*. 3ª ed. Lisbon: Edigoes Sílabo, 2003.

PIMENTA, G. - Professional motivation in situations of change: teaching in nursing. *Vital Signs*. N° 43 (2002), p. 19 - 21.

PIRES, A. L. - The new professional competencies. *Formar*. N° 10 (1994), p. 4-19.

POLIT, Denise F; HUNGLER, Bernadete P. - *Fundamentals of nursing research*. 3rd ed. Porto Alegre: Artes Médicas, 1995.

POLIT, Denise F; HUNGLER, Bernadete P. - *Investigación científica en ciencias de la salud*. 5.ª ed. México: Interamericana, 1997. p. 419-432.

PORTUGAL. Ministry of Health - *Health in Portugal: A strategy for the turn of the century*. Lisbon: Ministry of Health, 1997.

PORTUGAL. Ministério da Saúde, Departamento de Estudos e Planeamento de Saúde - *Inquérito Nacional de Saúde 1995/1997: regido norte*. Lisbon: Ministry of Health, 1997.

PORTUGAL. Ministério da Saúde, Direcgäo Recursos Humanos na Saúde - *Ensino de enfermagem: processos e percursos de formando - balando de um projecto*. Lisbon: Ministry of Health, 2000.

QUEIRÓS, A. A. - *Empathy and respect: central dimensions in the helping relationship*. Coimbra: Quarteto Editora, 1999.

QUIVY, R.; CAMPENHOUDT, L. V. - *Manual de investigacao em ciencias sociais*. 2nd ed. Lisbon: Gradiva, 1998.

REGO, A.; FERNANDES, C. - Inteligencia emocional: Desarrollo y validación de un instrumento de medida. *Revista Interamericana de Psicología*. Spain, in press.

ROSA, Maria Teresa S. - Study of the conditions for professional practice - Working Group. *Ordem dos Enfermeiros*. N° 14 (Oct. 2004), p. 12-14.

RUELA, Rosa - Behavior: A clever way out. *Visao*. (Nov. 1999), p. 119-120.

SAGEHOMME, Mme D. - *Por um trabalho melhor - guia de análise das condições de trabalho no meio hospitalar*. 3rd ed. Coimbra: FORMASAU - Formagäo e Saúde, 1997.

SALOVEY, P.; SLUYTER, D. J. - *Children's Emotional Intelligence*. Applications in education and everyday life. Rio de Janeiro: Campus, 1999.

SALOVEY, Peter; MAYER, John D.; CARUSO, David - The Positive Psychology of Emotional Intelligence. In SNYDER, C. R.; LOPEZ, S. J. - *The Handbook of Positive Psychology*. New York: Oxford University Press, 2002. p. 159-171.

SANTOS, Célia Samarina Vilaca de Brito - *Cognitive and Emotional*

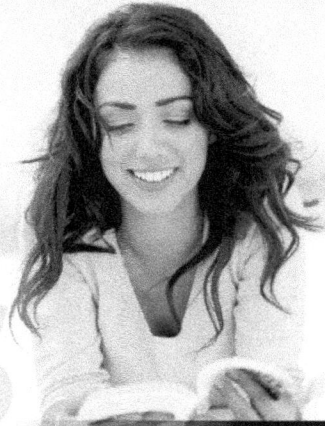

www.ingramcontent.com/pod-product-compliance
Lightning Source LLC
Chambersburg PA
CBHW021114210326
41598CB00017B/1442